AN ILLUSTRATED HANDBOOK
OF CHINESE QIGONG FORMS
FROM THE ANCIENT TEXTS

AN ILLUSTRATED HANDBOOK OF CHINESE QIGONG FORMS FROM THE ANCIENT TEXTS

Compiled by Li Jingwei and Zhu Jianping

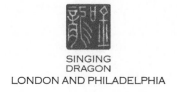

SINGING
DRAGON
LONDON AND PHILADELPHIA

This edition published in 2014
by Singing Dragon
an imprint of Jessica Kingsley Publishers
73 Collier Street
London N1 9BE, UK
and
400 Market Street, Suite 400
Philadelphia, PA 19106, USA

www.singingdragon.com

First published by Foreign Languages Press, Beijing, China, 2010

Copyright © Foreign Languages Press 2010, 2014

Printed digitally since 2016

Library of Congress Cataloging in Publication Data
A CIP catalog record for this book is available from the Library of Congress

British Library Cataloguing in Publication Data
A CIP catalogue record for this book is available from the British Library

ISBN 978 1 84819 197 6

PREFACE

Traditional Chinese health preservation has a long history, and consists of a broad variety of methods. According to "Gu Yue," as quoted in *Lü's Spring and Autumn Annals* of the pre-Qin period (c. 2100–221 BC), in the period of primitive society the ancient Chinese created the *daoyin* method, which combined physical and breathing exercises, for preventing and treating ailments of the joints and other diseases, and building up their health. "Ke Yi," as quoted in *The Book of Zhuangzi* of the Warring States Period (475–221 BC), spoke of the *daoyin* method for health preservation more explicitly, saying, "Breathe in and out to get rid of the old and take in the new; imitate a bear climbing and a bird spreading its wings to prolong life." The past several thousand years have witnessed a continuous development of Chinese health preservation methods, which became increasingly richer and diverse in content. Generally speaking, the health-preserving methods were kept in voluminous written records, with the exception of only a few in the form of pictures. These vivid pictures not only supplement the written descriptions, they are also precious cultural relics.

An *Illustrated Handbook of Chinese Qigong Forms from the Ancient Texts* is the result of the authors' meticulous work in collecting illustrations of Chinese health preservation methods (excluding those of the Taoist Neidan exercises for the time being) which appeared before the downfall of the last (Qing) Chinese dynasty in 1911, provided with captions taken from authentic written records. The pictures came from three sources: relics, books (including books on traditional Chinese and Tibetan medicine, and the Taoist Canon) and newly drawn pictures. Pictures from the first two sources are either reprinted or redrawn as closely as possible to resemble the originals. New illustrations follow the descriptions in ancient books which were unaccompanied by pictures.

The exercises appear in this book in chronological order, confirmed by archaeological and historical research. For instance, it was not until the Ming Dynasty (1368–1644) that illustrations of Hua Tuo's Five Animal Frolics appeared, although they had been recorded in the Three Kingdoms Period (220–280). Such an arrangement helps the reader follow the development of traditional Chinese health-preservation methods.

Textual research findings and a brief commentary are presented before each group of pictures with regard to the technique's emergence and evolution as well as notes on relevant sources. A caption from the original work follows, and a sentence-by-sentence explanation is provided to enable the readers to imitate the exercise.

It is our firm belief that this compilation of traditional Chinese health-preservation methods will be of benefit to all who are concerned with the health and happiness of oneself and others.

The editors
Beijing, 2010

PREFACE TO THE ENGLISH EDITION

With a history dating back to remote antiquity, Chinese studies on prolonging life through the cultivation of one's vital powers and health preservation have continuously developed, and their scientific basis has been refined and consolidated. Chinese history has witnessed a number of brilliant achievements in this regard, such as the *Picture of Daoyin Exercises* unearthed from the Mawangdui Tombs of the Han Dynasty (206 BC–220 AD), *qigong* of the Warring States Period (475–221 BC) demonstrated on the Inscription for Circulating *Qi* on a Jade Tablet, Five Animal Frolics created by physician Hua Tuo of the Three Kingdoms Period (220–280), the theory of Ge Hong of the Jin Dynasty (265–420) on the importance of moral cultivation for health preservation, and Tang Dynasty (618–907) physician and pharmacist Sun Simiao's proposal for combining quiescent *qigong* that gets rid of the old and takes in the new with the imitation of the movements of animals for health preservation, vitality cultivation and treatment of diseases of older age. In the later Song, Ming and Qing dynasties other scholars and physicians gradually improved and developed health-preserving theories. Extant Chinese books on these topics from the pre-Qin period (c. 2100–221 BC) to modern times number over 200, providing an invaluable data base for modern research in this respect.

Of these 200 titles, many contain graphic illustrations of the exercises, which helps the reader to grasp the key points. The illustrations not only have great practical value, but are also precious and delightful reminders of China's ancient culture. Based on the materials we had collected, we compiled the Chinese edition of this book several years ago, and it was well received. We were greatly encouraged, especially by Foreign Languages Press' decision to publish our book in English, German and French editions. We selected some color pictures on health preservation and have placed them in the center of the book. Although only one eighth of the original pictures, they can serve to give the readers an insight into the delicacy of some of the health-preserving illustrations. I hope that this book will enable readers to learn something of the vast amount of health-preserving knowledge acquired by the Chinese people through thousands of years, and find it beneficial for improving their own health and enriching their lives.

Li Jingwei
Beijing, 2010

CONTENTS

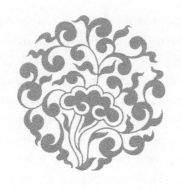

I

INSCRIPTION FOR THE CIRCULATION OF *QI* ON A JADE PENDANT

This inscription (see color illustrations in the center of the book) is a very precious cultural relic, being the oldest extant document relating to the theory of *qi*. Carved in the late Warring States Period (475–221 BC), it is a 12-faceted enclosed hollow cylinder. Each facet is inscribed with three characters. There are altogether 45 characters, including variants (see Fig 1.1). The object, previously the property of Li Mugong of Hefei, Anhui Province, is now in the collection of the Tianjin Museum. A rubbing of the inscription was first printed in *Yisheng*, and later in Luo Zhenyu's *A Collection of Ancient Bronze Inscriptions*. The inscription is reproduced here based on the TCM Yearbook 1983 and Luo's book.

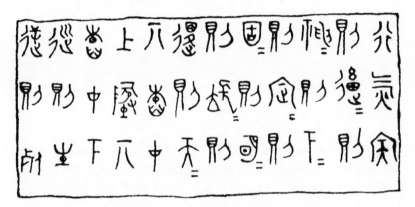

Figure 1.1
Inscription for the Circulation of *Qi* on a Jade Pendant

The gist of the inscription is: Take deep breaths to increase the storage of *qi* in the body, and direct the *qi* downward; fix the *qi* in the lower cavity with willpower so that the vital *qi* grows like sprouting seeds; send the *qi* upward back along the same route, and breathe it out slowly. People exercising by following this cycle from top to bottom will be healthy, while those who do otherwise will become sick and die.

II

DAOYIN EXERCISES

This picture appears on a colored silk painting 50 cm high and about 100 cm long, unearthed from Mawangdui Tomb Three of the Han Dynasty (206 BC–220 AD) in Changsha at the end of 1973. The picture shows 44 people in four rows, male and female, old and young, practicing *daoyin*, or physical and breathing exercises, in various postures and movements.

The painting is thought to have been put in the tomb no later than 168 BC, or the 12th year of the reign of Han Emperor Wendi.

In terms of the specific forms, this picture contains four aspects: 1. Empty-handed exercise, which most of the figures are engaged in; 2. Exercise with apparatus, four types of which can be seen, namely, plate, stick, ball and bag; 3. Deep breathing with the head raised; and 4. Meditation.

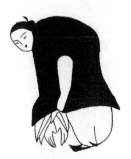

Figure 2.1

In terms of function, the exercises can be divided into health-preserving and therapeutic forms. The former imitate the movements of animals, such as mantis, bear and sparrow-hawk. Medical exercise is for treating diseases or serves as an aid to treating diseases. In most cases exercise for restoring the health of the organism involves the treatment of diseases through directing, such as directing deafness, the pathogenic factors in the flank and acute febrile and epidemic diseases.

For this book, 44 pictures were drawn based upon those on the silk painting.

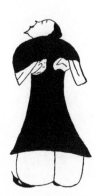

Figure 2.2

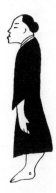

Figure 2.3

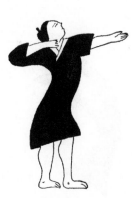

Figure 2.4

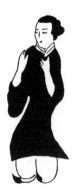

Figure 2.5

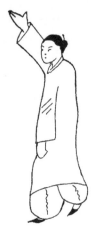

Figure 2.6
Bending for *Yin* Diseases

Stand straight. Twist to the right, and raise the right hand above the head leaving the left hand hanging by the side. This is a physical and breathing exercise for treating diseases in the *yin* meridians.

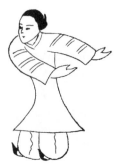

Figure 2.7

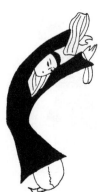

Figure 2.8
Mantis

Stand straight. Raise both hands above the head, and bend the waist toward the left. This is a physical and breathing exercise imitating the movement of a mantis.

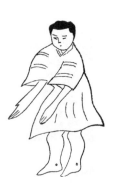

Figure 2.9

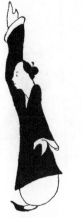

Figure 2.10

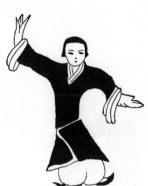

Figure 2.11

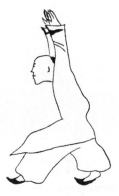

Figure 2.12

Figure 2.13
Costalgia

Stand straight. Move the
left foot one pace to the
right while holding the arms
horizontally and breathing
out slowly. This is a physical
and breathing exercise for
treating costalgia.

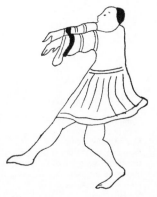

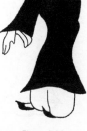

Figure 2.14

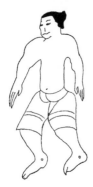

Figure 2.15
Hernia

Stand with the feet shoulder-width apart. Bend the head slightly forward and look downward without concentration. Let the arms hang down. Bend the knees slightly. This is a physical and breathing exercise for treating hernia.

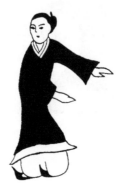

Figure 2.16

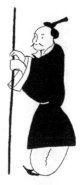

Figure 2.17

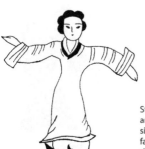

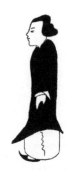

Figure 2.18
Abdominal Ailments

Stand straight. Stretch the arms horizontally to each side, with the right palm facing up and the left facing down. This is a physical and breathing exercise for treating diseases of the abdomen.

Figure 2.19

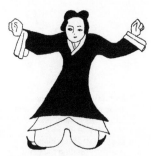

Figure 2.20
Deafness

Stand with the feet apart
and toes pointing outward.
Hunch the shoulders and
clench the fists. Assume
an expression of making a
great effort. This is a physical
and breathing exercise for
treating deafness.

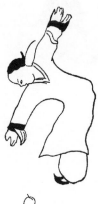

Figure 2.21

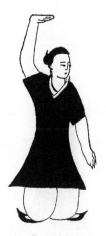

Figure 2.22
Tightness in Heart and Chest

Stand straight. Raise one arm
with the palm facing upward
while the other arm hangs
down. This is a physical
and breathing exercise for
treating tightness in the
heart and chest.

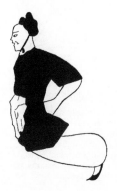

Figure 2.23
Knee Pain

Keep the upper body straight,
press both hands against the
small of the back. Try to bend
the knees while twisting the
body to the right. This is an
exercise for treating knee pain.

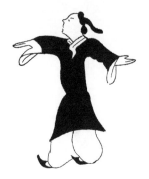

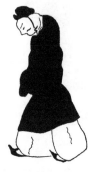

Figure 2.25
Flying Crane

Stand straight. Twist the body slightly to the right, and stretch the arms horizontally on each side. This is a physical and breathing exercise imitating the flight of a crane.

Figure 2.24
Pathogenic Factors in
the Flanks

Wearing a cap, bow the head. Place one foot in front of the other. Allow the arms to hang down, with one hand cupped in the other. This exercise is for eliminating pathogenic factors between the armpit and the waist.

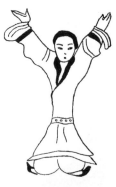

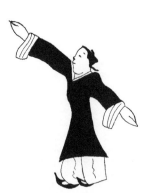

Figure 2.27
Flying Dragon

Stand straight with the feet shoulder-width apart. Stretch the arms upward in a V-shape, as if spreading the wings preparatory to flying. This is an imitation of a dragon flying.

Figure 2.26

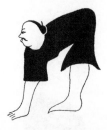

Figure 2.28
Ailments Resulting from Cold
Hands and Feet

Stoop, and touch the ground
with the palms while holding
the head up. This exercise is
for treating ailment resulting
from cold hands and feet.

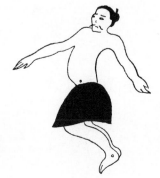

Figure 2.29
Neck Pain

Stand straight. Bend the
knees slightly, and hold the
arms some distance away
from the sides. Open the eyes
wide, and close the mouth.

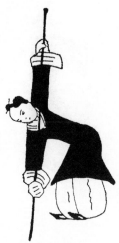

Figure 2.30
Regulating *Yin* and *Yang* with
a Staff

Stretch one arm upward and
the other downward, and
stoop while holding a staff
upright and placed against
the ground. This is a physical
and breathing exercise using
a staff as an aid to directing
the flow of *yin qi* and *yang qi*.

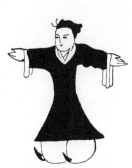

Figure 2.31
Sparrowhawk's Back

Stand straight. Stretch the
arms horizontally to the
sides. This is a physical and
breathing exercise imitating
the flight of a sparrowhawk
as if carrying the whole sky
on its back.

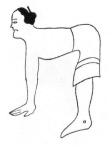

Figure 2.32
Bird Spreading its Wings

Stoop with a bare back to
imitate a bird spreading
its wings.

11

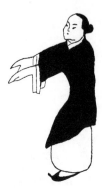

Figure 2.33

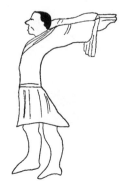

Figure 2.34
Breathing out with
Head Raised

Take a deep breath. Stretch
the arms upwards and
backwards while throwing
the chest forward and raising
the head. Breathe out.

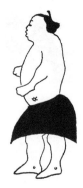

Figure 2.35
Expelling Internal Heat
by Imitating the Call of
a Macaque

Stand straight. Clench the
fists, and draw them to the
sides of the abdomen. Imitate
the call of a macaque. This
is for expelling Internal Heat
caused by deficiency of *yin*.

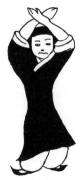

Figure 2.36
Acute Febrile and
Epidemic Diseases

Stand straight. Raise the
arms, and cross them in front
of the forehead.

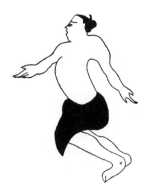

Figure 2.37
Regulating *Yin* and *Yang*

Kneel down. Stretch one
arm forwards and the other
backwards. This is a physical
and breathing exercise for
regulating the flow of *qi*
by learning the position
of Heaven and Earth, and
absorbing the *qi* of *yin* and
yang from Nature.

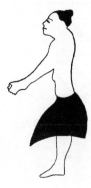

Figure 2.38

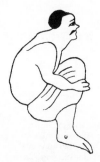

Figure 2.39
Expelling Pain
and Numbness

Squat and embrace the legs
with the arms. Draw the legs
up towards the breast. This
is a physical and breathing
exercise for expelling pains
and numbness caused by
wind, cold or damp.

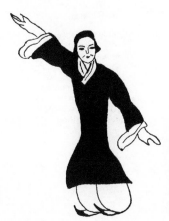

Figure 2.40
Monkey Breathing

Stand straight. Turn the body
a little to the right, and raise
the head. Stretch the right
arm forwards and upwards
and the left arm backwards
and downwards. This is
a physical and breathing
exercise imitating the way a
monkey howls.

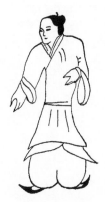

Figure 2.41
Bear Climbing

Stand straight. Raise the
arms to form a circle in front
of the chest, imitating the
way a bear climbs a tree.

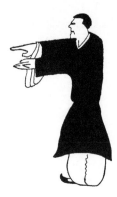

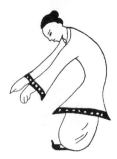

Figure 2.42
Dog Begging

Stand straight. Turn to the right, with the arms outstretched horizontally, in imitation of a dog standing on its hind legs and raising its head to beg.

Figure 2.43

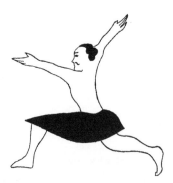

Figure 2.44
Zhan

Take a big step forward with the left foot, bending the left knee and straightening the right leg, with the body leaning slightly forward. Spread the arms outward and upward to imitate a *zhan* (bird of prey as recorded in ancient books) flying.

III

FIVE ANIMAL FROLICS

The Five Animal Frolics, a health-preserving method featuring rich physical movements, was compiled and created by Hua Tuo, a renowned physician of the Three Kingdoms Period (220–280). It is the fruit of the long-time practice of the ancient Chinese. *The Book of Zhuangzi*, written in the early Warring States Period (475–221 BC), records that the practice of *daoyin* exercises, such as "breathing in and out, getting rid of the old and taking in the new, imitating a bear climbing and a bird spreading its wings," had long been in existence. The *Picture of Daoyin Exercises* found in one of the Mawangdui Western Han Tombs in Changsha depicts people imitating a bear climbing, bird spreading its wings, monkey howling, etc. The book *Huainanzi*, also of the Western Han Dynasty, contains references to "bear climbing," "bird spreading its wings," "wild duck swimming," "monkey snatching food," "sparrowhawk glaring" and "tiger looking around" exercises, which were later referred to as the Six Animal Frolics. Drawing from and condensing the achievements of previous generations, Hua Tuo compiled the original Five Animal Frolics, namely five types of physical and breathing exercises imitating the movements of animals. They are "tiger frolic," "deer frolic," "bear frolic," "monkey frolic" and "bird frolic."

Besides his attainments in diagnosis, medicine, acupuncture and surgery, Hua Tuo was also proficient in techniques for preserving good health. He held the view that "It is advisable to do exercises, but not to go to extremes. Movement ensures good digestion of food and promotes blood circulation to guard against diseases. This is like a door hinge that never rusts." Hua Tuo therefore compiled and originated the Five Animal Frolics to sharpen the appetite and maintain health as well as cure disease. Wu Pu, a student of Hua Tuo, practiced these techniques, which preserved him from deafness and presbyopia and ensured him perfect teeth and a good appetite. He lived to over 90 years old.

Among the records of the specific methods of the Five Animal Frolics extant today, the earliest is the *Records on Cultivating the Character and Prolonging Life* compiled by Tao Hongjing of the Liang Dynasty (502–557). As it spread, the Five Animal Frolics was developed by numerous experts, who invented simple, complex, soft or rigid styles, and movements combined with breath and concentration control. For example, the Five Animal Frolics in the *Red Phoenix Marrow* by Zhou Lujing of the Ming Dynasty (1368–1644) are characterized by soft movements combined with breath and concentration control. They are much more advanced than the exercises that feature simple and enlarged movements recorded in the *Records on Cultivating the Character and Prolonging Life*. In the Ming Dynasty descriptions of the Five Animal Frolics were supplemented by illustrations. The illustrations in this book are based on those accompanying the Five Animal Frolics in *Red Phoenix Marrow* by Zhou Lujing.

Tiger Frolic

Stand with the head bowed. Clench the fists, and stretch the arms forward and downward like a fierce tiger about to pounce. Bend over, and raise the hands slowly as if lifting weights. Proceed until the body is upright. Take a deep breath into the abdomen. Direct *qi* upward and then downward, causing a thunderous roar in the abdomen. Repeat 15 times on each side. This exercise can promote the circulation of *qi* and blood to refresh the mind and eliminate diseases. (Figure 3.1)

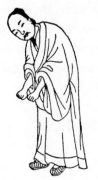

Figure 3.1

BEAR FROLIC

Stand and clench the fists. Move like a bear getting up sideways. Raise the right fist while leaving the left one hanging. Move the right foot back. Stand on the right foot. Lift the left foot. Coordinate the swinging movements of the left hand and the left foot. Repeat 15 times on each side. This causes sounds in the joints and stimulates *qi* and blood circulation in the flanks, which relaxes the muscles and joints, calms the mind and promotes blood circulation. (Figure 3.2)

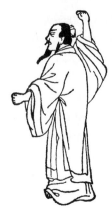

Figure 3.2

DEER FROLIC

Stand with the head bowed. Clench the fists, and imitate a deer turning its head to look at its tail. Then stand straight, and relax the shoulders. Stand on tiptoe, and then sink back onto the heels to shake the spine and the whole body. Repeat 15 times. This exercise can regulate *qi* and blood circulation throughout the body. (Figure 3.3)

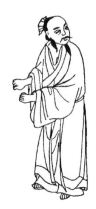

Figure 3.3

Monkey Frolic

Standing, imitate a monkey clasping a tree with its right hand and picking fruit with its left hand. Raise the head, and look at the left hand. Stand on the heel of the left foot. Lift and bend the right leg. Change to the opposite side. During this process concentrate the attention, hold the breath, click the teeth and swallow the saliva. Repeat 15 times on each side, or stop if perspiration occurs. (Figure 3.4)

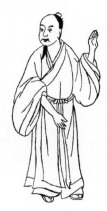

Figure 3.4

Bird Frolic

Standing, imitate a bird spreading its wings ready to take flight. Direct *qi* from the sacrum to the vertex. Raise the head, and clasp the hands in an arc over the forehead. Bend over, and separate the hands in imitation of a bird spreading its wings. Straighten the back, and clasp the hands over the forehead again. Repeat 15 times. This exercise can cure head diseases, raise *yin* in the kidneys and decrease heart fire. For women, it treats irregular menstruation and leukorrhea with bloody discharge, and eliminates various diseases. (Figure 3.5)

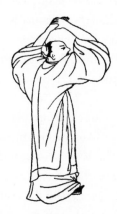

Figure 3.5

IV

SIX-CHARACTER FORMULA FOR TREATING DISEASES IN THE INTERNAL ORGANS

The six-character formula for treating diseases in the internal organs was first recorded in the Records of Cultivating the Character and Prolonging Life compiled by Tao Hongjing of the Liang Dynasty (502–557): "There are six ways of breathing out, namely *chui*, *hu*, *xi*, *he*, *xu* and *si*." The six-character formula is applied to treat various diseases. According to the book, "*Chui* disperses wind; *hu* removes heat; *xi* dispels upsets; *he* relieves tightness in the chest; *xu* eliminates staleness; and *si* relieves fatigue." In addition, "Distension in the chest caused by lung diseases can be released by *xu*." Thus, it is a series of exercises that cure diseases by breathing while reciting the formula silently.

Many new features were added to the six-character formula over the years. The Wise Master of the Sui Dynasty (581–618) paired the six characters with the internal organs: *he* with the heart, *hu* with the spleen, *si* with the lungs, *xu* with the liver and *xi* with the *sanjiao* (triple burner, three visceral cavities housing the internal organs). Later, physical movements were added to the exercises of breathing while reciting the six-character formula silently. Quiescent *qigong* was thus combined with dynamic *qigong*. The developed exercises were practiced as follows: For liver diseases, recite *xu* silently, and keep the eyes open; for lung diseases, recite *si* silently while raising two hands; for heart diseases, recite *he* with the hands crossed behind the head; for kidney diseases, recite *chui* while sitting on the ground with the knees clasped in the arms; for spleen diseases, recite *hu* with protruding lips; for diseases in the *sanjiao*, lie down and recite *xi*. Many works on the six-character formula with illustrations appeared, notable being *The Essence of Longevity* compiled by Xu Wenbi in 1771.

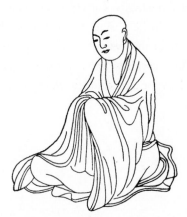

Figure 4.1
Six-Character Formula for Treating Diseases
of the Internal Organs

The Essence of Longevity, in eight volumes, discusses *qigong* and food therapy consecutively. The essays related to the six-character formula in "*Wushu* Exercises for Cultivation" in the first volume are illustrated with fresh drawings. The illustration on the previous page was reprinted from the 1775 block-printed edition of the *The Essence of Longevity*.

Steps: Every day between midnight and noon, sit still, click the teeth and swallow the saliva. Then recite the six characters *he, xu, hu, si, chui, xi* in an undertone, according to the rules for curing the diseases of the internal organs. Try to prolong the duration of recital of each character by protracting the breath. Among the six characters, *xu* and *xi* are easily confused. *Xu* is a labial syllable, while *xi* is a lingual syllable.

Points for attention: The six-character formula should be used only when one is ill, and discontinued as soon as one has recovered. For diseases of a particular internal organ, the corresponding character, instead of all the six characters, should be recited, so as to avoid harming the other healthy organs, i.e., *xu* for the liver, *he* for the heart, *si* for the lungs, *chui* for the kidneys, *hu* for the spleen and *xi* for the *sanjiao*. If several organs are affected, their corresponding characters can be applied together.

V

YIJINJING

Yijinjing is a type of dynamic *qigong* for limbering up the tendons. It is attributed to Bodhidharma, the founder of the Chan school of Buddhism in China, during the Northern and Southern Dynasties (420–589). As it is easy to learn it has long been a popular form of exercise. The first illustrated record of *Yijinjing* did not appear until the Song Dynasty (960–1279). Many styles emerged as it was spread and passed down, but the common practice at present is the set of exercises compiled by Pan Wei of the Qing Dynasty and included in his book *Major Methods of Health Preservation*. In the late Qing Dynasty, Zhou Shuguan renamed *Yijinjing* "the Twelve Wei Tuo Positions" in Volume 16 of his book *An Illustrated Book of Exercises to Benefit the Internal Organs–Promoting the Metabolism, Limbering Up the Tendons and Refreshing the Marrow*. The book contains 12 illustrations by Pan Wei. The following text and illustrations are from that book.

WEI TUO PRESENTING A PESTLE FORM 1

Stand straight, with the feet a fist's width apart. Throw out the chest, and tighten the abdomen. Hold the head erect, and look straight ahead. Keep the mouth closed, and let the tongue rest on the palate. Cup one hand in the other in front of the chest. With the eyes half-closed, inhale deeply through the nose and exhale through the mouth 30 times. (Figure 5.1)

WEI TUO PRESENTING A PESTLE FORM 2

Following the previous form, concentrate the weight on the balls of the feet. Extend the arms forwards, with the palms facing up, horizontally from the shoulders, and then to the sides. Breathe as in the previous exercise. Repeat 30 times. (Figure 5.2)

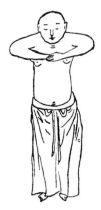

Figure 5.1
Wei Tuo Presenting a Pestle
Form 1

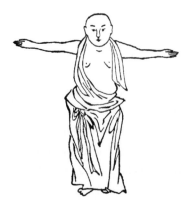

Figure 5.2
Wei Tuo Presenting a Pestle
Form 2

WEI TUO PRESENTING A PESTLE FORM 3

Raise the arms above the head, with the palms facing up. Straighten the elbows, and strain the palms as if holding the sky. The fingertips should point towards each other at a fist's distance apart. Straighten the knees, and stand on tiptoe, with eyes looking upward at the fingertips. Breathe as in the first two positions. Repeat 30 times. (Figure 5.3)

PLUCKING A STAR AND REPLACING IT WITH A DIPPER

Following the previous form, lower the arms to shoulder height. Bend the left elbow, and place the left forearm behind the back. Clutch the left shoulder blade. Turn the upper body leftward, keeping the lower part still. At the same time, raise the right hand above the head, with the palm facing the head. Look at the right palm and count from 1 to 30. Then turn the upper body to the front, and draw the right hand down to the chest. Move the right hand across the right part of the chest horizontally to the back to clutch the right shoulder blade. Move the left arm from back to the front of

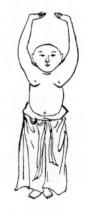

Figure 5.3
Wei Tuo Presenting a Pestle
Form 3

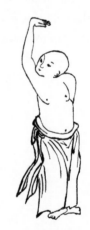

Figure 5.4
Plucking a Star and Replacing
it with a Dipper

25

the chest, and position it as the right arm mentioned above. Count from 1 to 30. Then draw both arms to the back, with the backs of the hands together. (Figure 5.4)

Pulling Nine Oxen Backwards by their Tails

Following the previous form, take a big step forward with the right foot to form a left bow step, bending the right leg and straightening the left one. Clench the right fist and raise it towards the upper right, with the elbow bent and the thumb facing the waist, as if lifting a huge weight. Clench the left fist in front of the chest, and bend the left elbow. Raise the upper left arm horizontal to the shoulder, and let the forearm dangle. Turn the head left slowly, and fix the eyes on the left fist. Breathe 30 times as in the previous positions. Then cross the fists in front of the lower abdomen and change to the right bow step. Repeat on the other side. Finally, cross the fists again in front of the lower abdomen. (Figure 5.5)

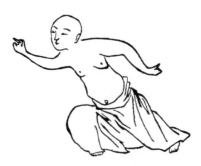

Figure 5.5
Pulling Nine Oxen Backwards
by their Tails

Extending the Claws and Spreading the Wings

Following the previous form, open the fists with palms outward, and draw the arms back to the sides. Raise the arms at the front to shoulder level. Stretch the arms forward, with the eyes focused on the hands. Straighten the legs, and apply the toes to the ground. Breathe 30 times as in the previous positions. Then clench the fists and bend the elbows. Draw the fists to the sides of the waist. (Figure 5.6)

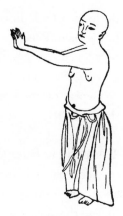

Figure 5.6
Extending the Claws and
Spreading the Wings

Nine Ghosts Drawing a Sword

Following the previous form, open the fists, raise your left hand upwards, and then place the left hand behind the back to clutch the left shoulder blade as in Plucking a Star and Replacing it with a Dipper. Raise the right hand over the head, to encircle the head with it. Turn the head to the left, with the four fingers of the right hand clinging to the groove along the edge of the left ear. Press the head against the hand. Extend the right elbow back as far as possible, and look straight forward. Breathe 30 times as in the previous positions. Hold the head erect, and move the right hand to the right side of the head. Stretch the right arm out horizontally to the right. Bend the right elbow, letting the right forearm dangle. Breathe 30 times as in the previous positions.

Repeat on the opposite side of the body. (Figure 5.7)

THREE ROCKS FALLING ON THE GROUND

Adopt the horse-riding stance, with the feet about one yard apart. Turn the toes slightly in, and the knees out. The knees should make approximately a right angle with the hip joints. Raise the hands to the level of the ears, and then move them downwards with the palms down, until they hang loosely by the thighs. Strain both hands with eyes and mouth wide open. Take 30 deep breaths. (Figure 5.8)

DRAGON EXTENDING ITS CLAWS

Lift the right hand to the side of the chest. Clench the fist, and turn the upper body to the left. Open the right fist, stretch the right hand with the palm up toward the front left, and stare at the right palm. Take 30 deep breaths. Then turn the right palm down, and lower the right arm without bending the elbow. Bend the waist

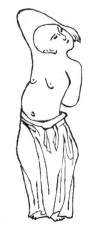

Figure 5.7
Nine Ghosts Drawing a
Sword

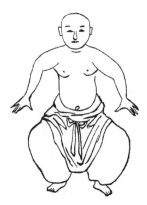

Figure 5.8
Three Rocks Falling on the
Ground

with the movement of the right hand. Move the right arm across the knees, and stretch it out and to the front. Straighten the waist, drawing the right fist to the right side of the chest. Turn the upper body to the right, and repeat the above movements on the other side. Take 30 deep breaths. Finally, return the body to an erect position, with the fists clenched at the sides. (Figure 5.9)

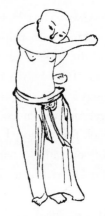

Figure 5.9
Dragon Extending its Claws

HUNGRY TIGER POUNCING ON ITS PREY

Take a big step forward with the right foot to form a right bow step, pressing the toes to the ground. Lean the upper body forward, with the fingers apart and slightly bent. Raise both hands with the palms up level with the top of the head. Move the hands down across the ears to the front of the body, and then lower them to the ground in front of the extended right foot. Press the ground with the fingers spread and the arms straight. Raise the head, and look forward like a tiger about to pounce on its prey. Take 30 deep breaths. Return the body to the erect position. Repeat the above movements on the other side, and then take 30 deep breaths. Finally, stand straight. (Figure 5.10)

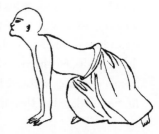

Figure 5.10
Hungry Tiger Pouncing on its Prey

Making a Deep Bow

Stand with the toes pointing outwards and the heels a fist's width apart. Clasp the back of the head with both hands, with the palms covering the ears. Bend at the waist and straighten the knees. Touch the knees with the head. Take 30 deep breaths. Return to the erect position with the hands still clasping the back of the head. (Figure 5.11)

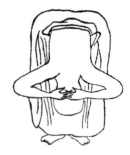

Figure 5.11
Making a Deep Bow

Raising the Tail

Move the hands, with the fingers interlaced, to the top of the head. Turn the palms up, and stretch the arms upwards. Then reverse the palms, and move them downwards along the chest. Straighten the knees, and bend the waist, pressing the palms on the toes. Hold the head up, and look straight ahead. Do not raise the heels. However, if you are unable to touch your toes, move the heels up and down in coordination with the breath. Take 30 deep breaths. Finally, return to the erect position, stretch the arms forward horizontally with the fingers interlaced and palms forward. (Figure 5.12)

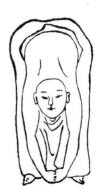

Figure 5.12
Raising the Tail

VI

TIANZHU MASSAGE

Tianzhu massage was first recorded in the *Essential Prescriptions for Emergencies Worth a Thousand Pieces of Gold (Precious Prescriptions for Emergencies)* by Sun Simiao (581–682), who was a noted physician and pharmacist in the Tang Dynasty. He decided to study medicine after surviving a sickly childhood. In 652 he composed the 30-volume *Essential Prescriptions for Emergencies Worth a Thousand Pieces of Gold*. Volume 27, titled *Character Cultivation*, includes experiences and methods passed down through the ages in the sphere of health preservation, such as living habits, massage therapy, breathing exercises, diet therapy and sanitation. The volume embraces nearly every aspect of traditional Chinese health-preservation culture, which Sun Simiao developed by expounding on those aspects from his own point of view. He advocated combining quiescent *qigong* that gets rid of the old and takes in the new with dynamic *qigong* imitating the movements of animals, such as the agile and steady climbing method of the bear and the vigilance of the sparrowhawk. He attached importance to regularity and moderation in daily life, including diet, temperament, housing conditions, and so on, as well as a combination of health-preserving exercises and treatment of diseases of old age. Thus Sun Simiao developed health preservation into a science consisting of both theory and practice.

"Massage Methods" in Volume 27, *Character Cultivation*, includes two sets of dynamic exercises—Tianzhu massage and Laozi massage (see Chapter VII). It is said that Tianzhu massage was a set of massage exercises called "Brahman massage" (Brahmanic gymnastics) with 18 positions. Tianzhu is the Chinese name for ancient India, and Brahmanism is one of the ancient Indian religions. However, no solid evidence has been found to bear out the Indian origin of this set of techniques. Many books on health preservation thereafter incorporated "Brahman massage," such as the *Seven Slips of a Cloudy Satchel* of the Song Dynasty and *Eight Essays on Health Preservation* of the Ming Dynasty. Sun Simiao claimed that practicing the set three times a day could enable elderly people to "get rid of all diseases and fatigue, run as fast as a steed, prolong life, sharpen the appetite and eyesight, and become agile in one month." The following 18 illustrations are based on descriptions in the *Essential Prescriptions for Emergencies Worth a Thousand Pieces of Gold*.

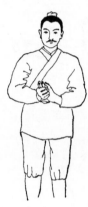

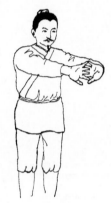

Figure 6.1

Rub the hands as if washing them.

Figure 6.2

Interlace the fingers, and push them forward, with the palms outward. Then turn the palms inward and draw the hands back to the chest. Repeat.

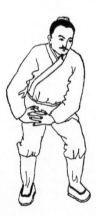

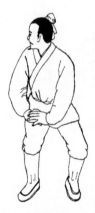

Figure 6.4

Place one hand over the other, and press on the right thigh. Turn the upper body rightwards slowly. Repeat on the other side.

Figure 6.3

Interlace the fingers, and press them on each thigh successively.

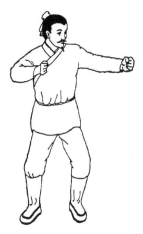

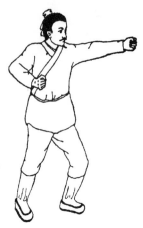

Figure 6.5

Position the arms as if pulling on a fully extended bow, with the left hand holding the bow and the right holding the string. Repeat on the other side.

Figure 6.6

Clench the fists, and pound the air, alternating the fists.

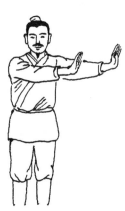

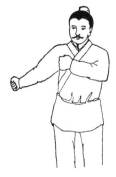

Figure 6.8

Clench the fists. Beat the right chest with the left fist while swinging the right hand backwards. Repeat on the other side. This is a method of expanding the chest.

Figure 6.7

Stretch both arms to one side as if pushing a large stone. Repeat on the other side.

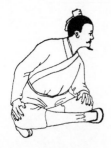

Figure 6.9

Cross the legs naturally, and sit on the ground. Bend the upper body and lean to one side as if a mountain is toppling. Repeat on the other side.

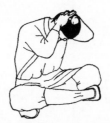

Figure 6.10

Clutch the nape of the neck with both hands, and turn the head left and right over the thighs, with the head bent forward and low. This is a method of limbering up the head.

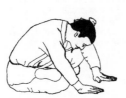

Figure 6.11

Sit on the ground cross-legged. Press the hands against the ground, and bend the upper body forward. Huddle with the back curved. Raise the arms three times.

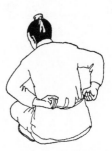

Figure 6.12

Beat the back with the fists.

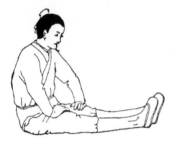

Figure 6.13

Sit steadily on the ground
with the legs straight out.
Stretch the legs forward
alternately.

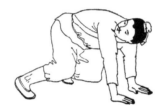

Figure 6.14

Press the hands against the
ground, and turn the head
backwards toward the upper
right. Open the eyes wide,
like a tiger glaring at its prey.
Repeat on the other side.

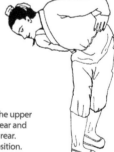

Figure 6.15

Stand straight. Bend the upper
body toward the left rear and
then toward the right rear.
Return to the erect position.
Do this exercise three times.

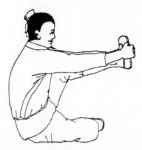

Figure 6.16

With the fingers interlaced, put
tension on the raised left foot.
Repeat with the right foot.

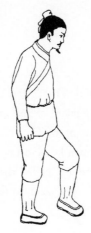

Figure 6.17

Standing, stamp the feet
alternately.

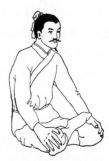

Figure 6.18

Sit with the left foot placed
on the right knee and the
right foot placed on the left
knee. Then press the knees
down with the hands.

VII

LAOZI MASSAGE

Laozi massage was first recorded in the "Massage Techniques" in *Character Cultivation* of the *Essential Prescriptions for Emergencies Worth a Thousand Pieces of Gold* complied by Sun Simiao of the Tang Dynasty (see Chapter VI). The *Eight Essays on Health Preservation* by Gao Lian of the Ming Dynasty also includes Laozi Massage, where it is called the "Supreme Way Massage." The following 35 illustrations are based on those in this work. Taishang is the posthumous title of Laozi.

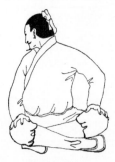

Figure 7.1

Press the hands on the thighs, and turn the upper body to the left and to the right. Repeat 21 times.

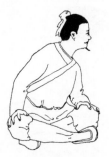

Figure 7.2

Press the hands on the thighs, and turn the shoulders to the left and to the right. Repeat 14 times.

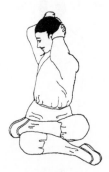

Figure 7.3

Place the hands behind the head, and turn the waist to the left and to the right. Repeat 14 times.

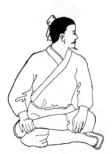

Figure 7.4

Turn the head to the left and to the right. Repeat 14 times.

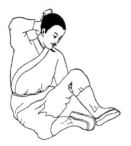

Figure 7.5

Place the right hand behind the head, and hold the left leg under the knee with the left hand to form a triangle with the leg. Repeat on the other side.

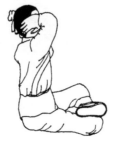

Figure 7.6

Place the hands on the sides of the head and raise the head three times.

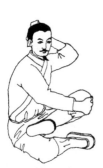

Figure 7.7

Place the left hand on the back of the head. Using the right hand, raise the left knee, with the lower leg horizontal. Repeat on the other side.

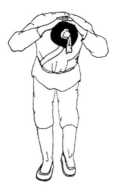

Figure 7.8

In a standing position, place the hands behind the head, and bow from the waist three times, then stamp the feet.

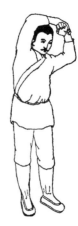

Figure 7.9

Hold the wrist of one hand with the other hand over the head, and pull to the left and to the right. Repeat three times on each side.

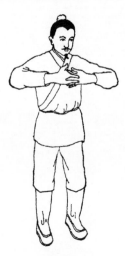

Figure 7.10

With the fingers interlaced, draw the hands towards the chest, palms inward. Then push forward with the palms outward. Repeat three times. Then draw and push the hands with the palms inward three times.

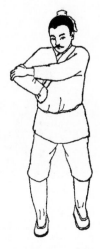

Figure 7.11

Bend the right wrist and press it against the right ribs. Pull the right elbow with the left hand. Repeat three times on each side.

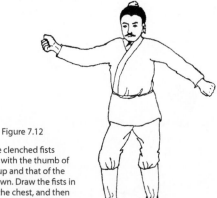

Figure 7.12

Raise the clenched fists laterally, with the thumb of one fist up and that of the other down. Draw the fists in front of the chest, and then stretch the arms backwards. Repeat three times.

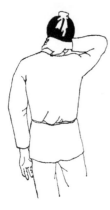

Figure 7.13

Place the right hand on the nape of the neck, and pull the neck to the right three times. Repeat on the other side.

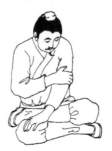

Figure 7.14

Seated cross-legged, press the left hand on the right knee. Pull the left elbow with the right hand, and then press the right hand on the left hand. Change to the other side, and repeat three times on each side.

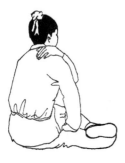

Figure 7.15

Seated cross-legged, stroke the right shoulder from above with the left hand. Repeat on the other side.

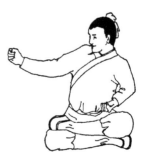

Figure 7.16

Seated cross-legged, form hollow fists and punch forward three times.

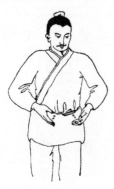

Figure 7.17

Standing, shake the hands outward, inward and downward three times each.

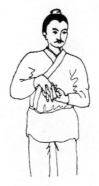

Figure 7.18

Interlace the fingers, and twist the wrists seven times on each side.

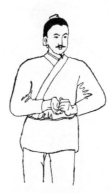

Figure 7.19

Rub and wring the fingers ten times.

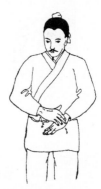

Figure 7.20

Straighten the palms and shake one with the other back and forth three times on each side.

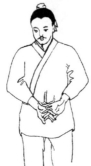

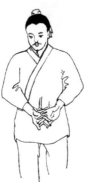

Figure 7.21

Interlace the fingers, with the hands back to back, and move the hands up and down many times to exercise the elbows. Repeat for ten breaths if this exercise is done on its own.

Figure 7.22

Interlace the fingers, and place the hands over the head with the palms facing up. Stretch the arms upwards and press downwards three times each.

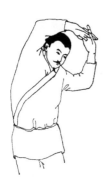

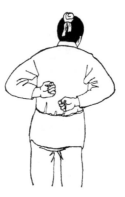

Figure 7.23

With the fingers interlaced and the hands over the head with the palms down, stretch the ribs left and right ten times each.

Figure 7.24

Beat the upper back and lower back three times each with the backs of the fists.

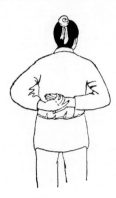

Figure 7.25

Hold one hand in the other at the back, and stroke the spine up and down three times.

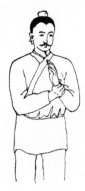

Figure 7.26

Grasp the inner left wrist in the right palm and shake the left hand outwards. Repeat three times on each side.

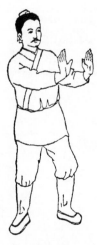

Figure 7.27

Hold the palms upright and facing outwards. Push them forwards three times.

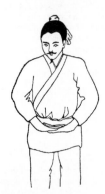

Figure 7.28

Interlock the fingers horizontally, with the palms down. Press the hands downwards three times.

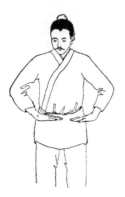

Figure 7.29

Align the hands horizontally, palms down and the fingertips facing each other. Lift and lower the hands together three times. Pat the body from top to bottom until the hands get warm to cure the problem of cold hands.

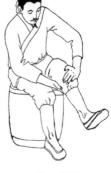

Figure 7.30

Seated on a stool, cross the left leg over the right one, and insert the right hand between the knees. Stroke the lower left leg with the left hand from top to bottom three times. Repeat on the other side.

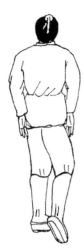

Figure 7.31

Stand on the left foot, and lift the right heel from the ground. Turn the right ankle clockwise and then anti-clockwise three times each. Repeat with the left foot.

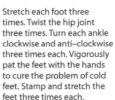
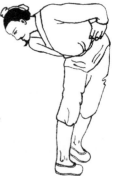

Figure 7.32

Stretch each foot three times. Twist the hip joint three times. Turn each ankle clockwise and anti–clockwise three times each. Vigorously pat the feet with the hands to cure the problem of cold feet. Stamp and stretch the feet three times each.

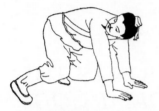

Figure 7.33

Crouch on the ground like a tiger. Turn the head to look back over the left and right shoulders three times respectively.

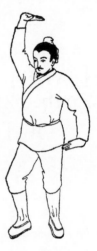

Figure 7.34

Stretch the right arm up, with the palm up as if holding up the sky while pressing the left palm down. Repeat three times on each side alternately.

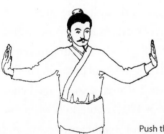

Figure 7.35

Push the hands to the sides three times with erect palms, as if toppling mountains. Bend the waist as if carrying a mountain on the back while pulling the hands three times as if pulling a tree.

VIII

HEALTH PRESERVATION IN THE *FOUR-VOLUME MEDICAL CODE* OF TIBETAN MEDICINE

The *Four-Volume Medical Code* was compiled by leading Tibetan medical practitioner Yutog Nyingma Yundain Goinbo (708–?) in the latter half of the eighth century. The extant version is the one revised by Yutog's descendant Yutog Sama Yundain Goinbo in the 11th century. Volume 1 is the *General Introduction*; Volume 2, *Exposition*, deals with the human anatomy, etiology, pathology, symptoms and principles for treatment; Volume 3, *Recipes*, addresses the classification of diseases and corresponding treatments; Volume 4, *Supplement*, deals with diagnosis by feeling the pulse and examining the urine, pharmacology and techniques of preparing herbal medicines, moxibustion, bloodletting and external application of medicine. In the late 17th century, Sangye Gyatso (1653–1705) and others wrote the *Annotations to the Four-Volume Medical Code*, thoroughly annotating and developing the *Four-Volume Medical Code*. Later, Sangye Gyatso and others compiled *The Complete Four-Volume Medical Code Wall Chart Series* according to the *Annotations to the Four-Volume Medical Code* and the wall charts drawn by the northern and southern schools of Tibetan medicine in the 15th century. The album consists of 79 colored pictures, among which the 54th and 55th wall charts (see the color illustrations in the center of the book) concern health preservation. The following 24 pictures were copied from *The Complete Four-Volume Medical Code Wall Chart Series*.

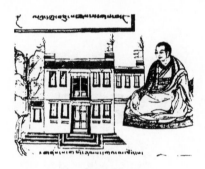

Figure 8.1

Keep the house comfortable and clean.

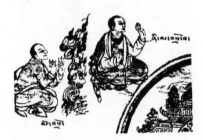

Figure 8.2

Keep warm and bask in the sunshine often.

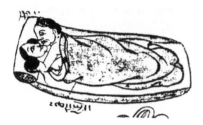

Figure 8.3

Moderate your sex life.

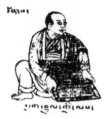

Figure 8.4

Avoid heavy lifting.

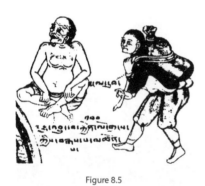

Figure 8.5

Seniors should not overwork themselves.

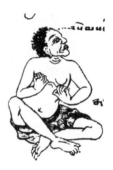

Figure 8.6

Do not overstrain the heart.

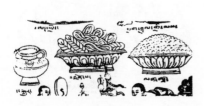

Figure 8.7

Minimize intake of salt, raw
and cold food.

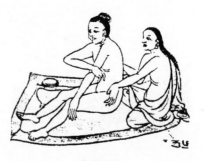

Figure 8.8

Keep the body and
feet clean.

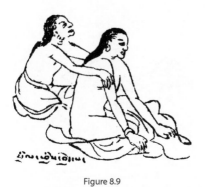

Figure 8.9

Smear cream on the body
evenly and wipe off dirt.

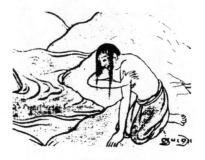

Figure 8.10

Bathe often.

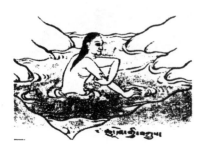

Figure 8.11

Bathe in hot springs.

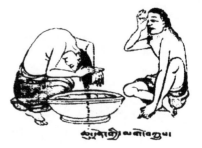

Figure 8.12

Wash the hair in warm water.

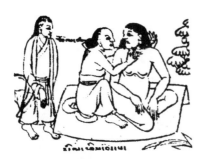

Figure 8.13

Do exercises, and wipe the
body often.

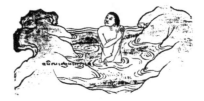

Figure 8.14

Bathe in cold water often.

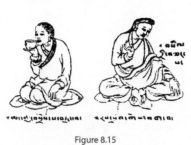

Figure 8.15

Drink alcohol in moderation,
and wear thin clothes.

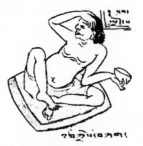

Figure 8.16

Avoid excessive hunger.

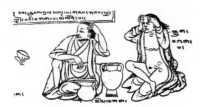

Figure 8.17

Avoid thirst and suppression
of vomiting.

Figure 8.18

Do not hold back a sneeze or
a yawn.

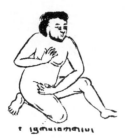

Figure 8.19

Breathe naturally.

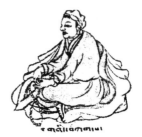

Figure 8.20

Get enough sleep.

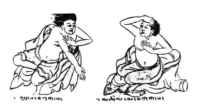

Figure 8.21

Spit out sputum immediately.

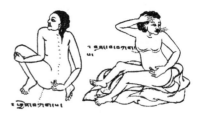

Figure 8.22

Do not delay the breaking of
wind or defecation.

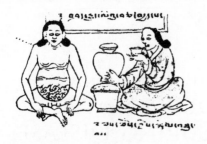

Figure 8.23

Maintain a moderate diet.

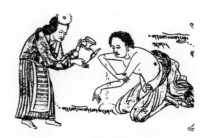

Figure 8.24

Pay attention to hygiene.

IX

TWENTY-FOUR-SEASONAL-DIVISION-POINTS SEATED EXERCISES FOR CURING DISEASES

The Twenty-four-Seasonal-Division-Points Seated Exercises for Curing Diseases are said to have been created by Chen Tuan, who was an expert on health preservation in the Song Dynasty. Illustrations for the exercises appeared in the Ming Dynasty. Volume 2 of the three-volume *Immortals' Methods for Achieving Longevity* (*Wanshou Xianshu*) compiled by Luo Hongxian of the Ming Dynasty incorporates the captioned "Illustrations for the Seasonal Seated Exercises for Curing Diseases," but these are ancient and illegible. Pictures and captions in Volume 4 of the *Essentials of Health Preservation of China and Other Countries*, compiled by Zheng Guanying of the Qing Dynasty, are relatively clear. Therefore, the following pictures were reprinted from the 1893 block-printed edition of the latter.

Zheng Guanying (1842–1921) was born in Xiangshan (today's Zhongshan), Guangdong Province. A sickly child, Zheng was impelled to study techniques of health preservation. He considered good living habits, a moderate diet, few worldly desires, tranquillity of mind through cultivation of *qi*, light, heat, air, water, diet and exercise all to be essential elements for health preservation. Zheng said that he had "compiled the essentials of health preservation recorded by great thinkers of the past, my teachers and friends, into two volumes, and instructions on food choices in daily life in one volume, and *wushu*, massage and *daoyin* exercises in another volume. The four volumes are put together under the title *Essentials of Health Preservation of China and Other Countries*." Volume four contains illustrations for Chen Tuan's Twenty-four-Seasonal-Division-Points Seated Exercises, *yijinjing*, Eight-section Brocade Seated Exercises and Chen Tuan's sleep exercises, and is a valuable reference work.

The twenty-four seasonal division points are used as a way of marking the changes in season and weather in the solar year, which is divided according to the Chinese lunar calendar. At the most, one or two days of discrepancy may appear in the date of the points between two successive years in the solar calendar. The twenty-four seasonal division points are: 1.Beginning of Spring (February 5); 2. Rain Water (February 19); 3. Waking of Insects (March 5); 4. Vernal Equinox (March 20); 5. Pure Brightness (April 5); 6. Grain Rain (April 20); 7. Beginning of Summer (May 5); 8. Grain Budding (May 21); 9. Grain in Ear (June 6); 10. Summer Solstice (June 21); 11. Slight Heat (July 7); 12.Great Heat (July 23); 13. Beginning of Autumn (August 7); 14. Limit of Heat (August 23); 15. White Dew (September 8); 16. Autumnal Equinox (September 23); 17. Cold Dew (October 8); 18. Descent of Frost (October 23); 19. Beginning of Winter (November 7); 20. Slight Snow (November 22); 21. Great Snow (December 7); 22. Winter Solstice (December 21); 23. Slight Cold (January 6); 24. Great Cold (January 21).

The Twenty-four-Seasonal-Division-Points Seated Exercises are a method of preserving health and treating diseases according to the changes in the season and weather. Each division point refers to a period of time rather than a particular day. For example, the Beginning of Spring refers to the period of time around February 5. January, February...December in the titles of the exercises, are all Chinese lunar months.

Seated Exercise at the Beginning of Spring, February

Application: Rheumatic pains, cold, distension of *qi*, and pain in the neck, behind the ears, and in the shoulders, arms, back and elbows.

Steps: Every night between 11 pm and 3 am sit cross-legged. Place one hand over the other, and press on one thigh. Turn the upper body to the right, and rotate the head, with the eyes looking toward the upper rear right. Stretch the neck, and keep this position for a few seconds. Then turn the upper body slowly to the left, and repeat the movements above on the left side. Repeat 15 times on each side. Click the teeth 36 times. Gargle with the saliva nine times and then swallow a mouthful of saliva in three gulps. Imagine sending the saliva to the *dantian* (or the pubic region). It is believed that your natural life energy is stored there. Gargle with the saliva three times, and swallow the gathered saliva in nine gulps. Inhale through the nose and exhale through the mouth in slow, long, even and deep breaths. Each inhalation and exhalation are counted as one breath. Repeat 36 times. The exercise can also be done in the early morning. So can the other exercises below.

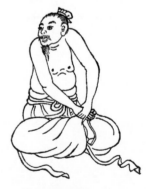

Figure 9.1
Seated Exercise at the
Beginning of Spring, February

Seated Exercise at Rain Water, February

Application: Stagnant harmful factors in the main and collateral channels (meridians) of the *sanjiao*, swollen and dry throat, vomiting, hiccupping, numb throat, deafness, excessive sweating and sharp pains in the canthus and cheeks.

Steps: Every night between 11 pm and 3 am sit cross-legged. Place one hand over the other, and press on one thigh. Turn the upper body and the head to the left. Lean the head leftward, and keep this position for a few seconds. Then change to the right side. Repeat 15 times on each side. Finally, click the teeth, gargle with the saliva and swallow. Inhale and exhale as in the previous form.

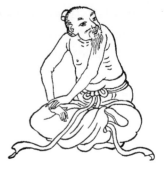

Figure 9.2
Seated Exercise at Rain Water,
February

Seated Exercise at Waking of Insects, March

Application: Stagnant harmful factors in the waist, spine, spleen and stomach, jaundiced eyes and dry mouth, nose and gum bleeding, intermittent headaches and swollen face, numb and hoarse throat, dim eyes and photophobia, dull sense of smell and lumps throughout the body.

Steps: Every morning between 1 am and 5 am sit cross-legged and clench the fists. Turn the head to the left and right slowly four times each. Bend the elbows and raise the forearms to chest level, with the palms down and the fingers bent naturally. Pull the elbows backward simultaneously. Repeat 30 times. Finally, click the teeth, gargle with the saliva and swallow. Inhale and exhale as in the previous form.

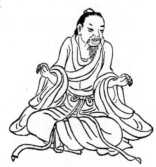

Figure 9.3
Seated Exercise at Waking of
Insects, March

SEATED EXERCISE AT VERNAL EQUINOX, MARCH

Application: Stagnant harmful factors in the main and collateral channels (meridians) of the chest, shoulders and back, physical weakness, painful teeth, swollen neck, fierce cold with hot swellings, deafness and ringing in the ears, heat behind the ears, painful shoulders and arms, swollen skin and itching.

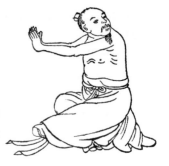

Figure 9.4
Seated Exercise at Vernal
Equinox, March

Steps: Every morning between 1 am and 5 am, sit cross-legged. Lift the hands along the sides to the armpits, with the palms up. Turn the palms inward, and push the arms forward horizontally at shoulder width, with the fingers pointing up. At the same time, turn the head to the left. Then draw back the hands to the armpits, and turn the face to the front. Push out the hands as above and turn the head to the right. Repeat 42 times on each side. Finally, click the teeth, gargle with the saliva and swallow. Inhale and exhale as in the previous form.

Seated Exercise at Pure Brightness, April

Application: Stagnant harmful factors in the waist, spine, spleen and stomach, heat around the ears, bitter cold, deafness, sore throat, pains in the neck, shoulders and arms and weak waist.

Steps: Every morning between 1 am and 5 am sit cross-legged. Position the hands as if drawing a bow. Repeat 56 times on each side. Finally, click the teeth, gargle with the saliva and swallow. Inhale and exhale as in the previous form.

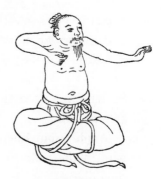

Figure 9.5
Seated Exercise at Pure Brightness, April

Seated Exercise at Grain Rain, April

Application: Lumps and gores in the spleen and stomach, jaundiced eyes, nose bleed, swollen cheeks and jaw, painful swollen upper outside arms and hot palms.

Steps: Every morning between 1 am and 5 am sit cross-legged. Raise the right arm, with the palm up and fingertips pointing left, as if holding the sky. Bend the left arm in a right angle, and place the forearm horizontally in front of the chest, with the fingers bent naturally and the palm inward. Turn the head left, with the eyes looking front left. Change to the other side.

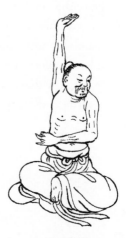

Figure 9.6
Seated Exercise at Grain Rain, April

Repeat 35 times on each side. Finally, click the teeth, gargle with the saliva and swallow. Inhale and exhale as in the previous form.

SEATED EXERCISE AT THE BEGINNING OF SUMMER, MAY

Application: Rheumatism, swelling and pain in the main and collateral channels (meridians), convulsions in the arms and elbows, swollen armpit, hot palms and hysteria.

Steps: Every day between 3 am and 7 am bend both legs. Lay one leg on the ground, and embrace the knee of the other with the fingers interlaced. Push with the knee and pull with the hands for two or three seconds. Repeat with each leg 35 times alternately. Finally, click the teeth, gargle with the saliva and swallow. Inhale and exhale as in the previous form.

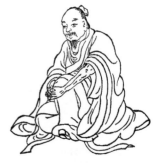

Figure 9.7
Seated Exercise at the
Beginning of Summer, May

SEATED EXERCISE AT GRAIN BUDDING, MAY

Application: Stagnant harmful factors in the lungs, distended chest and flanks, irregular or rapid heart beat, flushed face and nose, jaundiced eyes, heartburn and hot palms.

Steps: Every morning between 3 am and 7 am sit cross-legged. Press on the calf with the left hand and raise the right hand as if holding the sky, with the fingertips pointing left. Change to the other side. Repeat 15 times on each side. Finally, click the teeth, gargle with the saliva and swallow. Inhale and exhale as in the previous form.

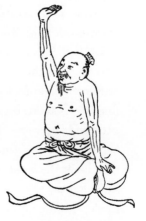

Figure 9.8
Seated Exercise at Grain Budding, May

STANDING EXERCISE AT GRAIN IN EAR, JUNE

Application: Physical weakness in the waist and kidneys, dry throat, stomachache, jaundiced eyes, pain in the flanks, frequent drinking and urination, hysteria, panic, forgetfulness, coughing and vomiting, depletion of *qi*, heat throughout the body and pain in the thighs, melancholia, headache and neck pains, and flushed face.

Steps: Every morning between 3 am and 7 am stand with the feet apart at shoulder width. Raise the hands to chest level, with the palms upward, and then turn the palms outward. Straighten the arms, with the palms upward and fingertips pointing back. Stick out the abdomen, and bend backwards. Look at the backs of the hands. Keep this position for a few seconds, and then lower the hands gradually to hang by the sides. Repeat 35 times. Finally, click the teeth, gargle with the saliva and swallow. Inhale and exhale as in the previous form.

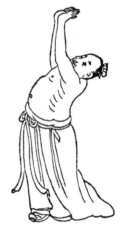

Figure 9.9
Standing Exercise at Grain in Ear, June

SEATED EXERCISE AT SUMMER SOLSTICE, JUNE

Application: Rheumatism, pains in the wrists, ankles, knees, shoulders, arms, kidneys, waist and back, aching hot palms, fatigue and weakness.

Steps: Every morning between 3 am and 7 am squat. Stretch the arms forward, and interlace the fingers with the palms facing inward. Push against the hands with the right foot. Keep this position for two or three seconds, and then change to the left leg. Repeat 35 times on each side. Finally, click the teeth, gargle with the saliva and swallow. Inhale and exhale as in the previous form.

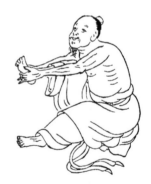

Figure 9.10
Seated Exercise at Summer Solstice, June

SEATED EXERCISE AT SLIGHT HEAT, JULY

Application: Rheumatism in the legs, knees, waist and hipbone, dry throat, asthma and coughing, distended lower abdomen, hemiplegia, amnesia, rectocele, feeble wrists, moodiness.

Steps: Every morning between 1 am and 5 am prop the hands on the ground at the back, with straightened elbows and fingertips pointing backwards. Stretch the left foot forward, with the heel touching the ground. Bend the right leg, pressing the thigh on the calf. With the eyes fixed on the toes of the left foot, shift the center of gravity backwards and then forwards. Repeat 15 times on each side. Finally, click the teeth, gargle with the saliva and swallow. Inhale and exhale as in the previous form.

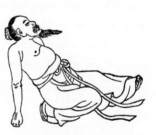

Figure 9.11
Seated Exercise at Slight
Heat, July

67

SEATED EXERCISE AT GREAT HEAT, JULY

Application: Rheumatism in the head, neck, chest and back, coughing, asthma, distended chest, pain in the arms, shoulders, back or above the navel, hot palms, frequent urination, numbness and pain in the skin, chill and fever.

Steps: Every morning between 1 am and 5 am sit cross-legged. Prop the fists on the ground in front of the legs, with the thumb sides of the fists facing each other. Straighten the arms at shoulder width apart, and shift the center of gravity forward. Bend the upper body forward, and turn the head to the left, with the eyes wide open glaring to the upper left. Then shift the center of gravity backwards, and turn the face to the front. Shift the center of gravity forwards again, and turn the head to the right, with the eyes wide open and glaring to the upper right. Repeat 15 times on each side. Finally, click the teeth, gargle with the saliva and swallow. Inhale and exhale as in the previous form.

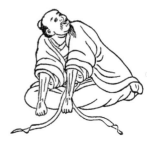

Figure 9.12
Seated Exercise at Great
Heat, July

Seated Exercise at the Beginning of Autumn, August

Application: Physical weakness, depletion of qi, stagnant qi in the waist and back, bitter taste in the mouth, frequent sighing, pains in the chest and flanks, inability to turn over in bed, pale face, hot outward sides of feet, headache, aching jaw and eye sockets, swollen armpits, and painful and swollen shoulder sockets.

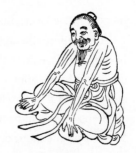

Figure 9.13
Seated Exercise at the
Beginning of Autumn, August

Steps: Every morning between 1 am and 5 am sit cross-legged. Bend the upper body forward, and prop it on the arms straightened and shoulder-width apart. Draw the chest inward, and huddle the body. Holding the breath, stretch the body upward, and shift the center of gravity forward. Keep this position for a while, and then return to the beginning position. Finally, click the teeth, gargle with the saliva and swallow. Inhale and exhale as in the previous form.

Seated Exercise at Limit of Heat, August

Application: Rheumatism, painful shoulders, back and chest, pain in the gallbladder meridian and in the joints, shortness of breath, coughing, and stagnant *qi* in the chest and back.

Steps: Every morning between 1 am and 5 am sit on the ground. Point the head toward the rear upper left, and then toward the rear upper right. Meanwhile, beat the lower back with the back of the hollow fists. Beat six times for every turn of the head. Turn the head to each side 35 times. Finally, click the teeth, gargle with the saliva and swallow. Inhale and exhale as in the previous form.

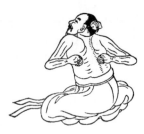

Figure 9.14
Seated Exercise at Limit of Heat, August

Seated Exercise at White Dew, September

Application: Rheumatic pains and stagnant *qi* in the lower back meridian, chill, disturbed by people and fire, frightened at the sound of water, malaria, sweating, nosebleed, ulcerated lips, swollen neck, numb throat and inability to speak, and vomiting.

Steps: Every morning between 1 am and 5 am sit cross-legged. Press each hand on the thigh on

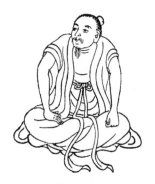

Figure 9.15
Seated Exercise at White Dew, September

the same side, and turn the head to the left and right slowly 15 times each side. Finally, click the teeth, gargle with the saliva and swallow. Inhale and exhale as in the previous form.

SEATED EXERCISE AT AUTUMNAL EQUINOX, SEPTEMBER

Application: Rheumatism, ascites, swollen and painful kneecaps, distended chest and abdomen, pain in the outer thighs and shins, enuresis, morbid thirst, stomach chill and breathlessness.

Steps: Every morning between 1 am and 5 am sit cross-legged. Press the hands over the ears with the fingertips pointing to each other. Bend the upper body slowly leftwards as far as possible, and then to the right. Repeat 15 times on each side. Finally, click the teeth, gargle with the saliva and swallow. Inhale and exhale as in the previous form.

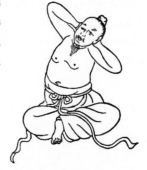

Figure 9.16
Seated Exercise at Autumnal
Equinox, September

SEATED EXERCISE AT COLD DEW, OCTOBER

Application: Cold and rheumatism in the flank and armpit meridians, distension in the head and neck, back pains, jaundiced and tearing eyes, nosebleed and cholera.

Steps: Every morning between 1 am and 5 am sit cross-legged. Raise the hands slowly to the front of the chest, with the palms up and the fingertips pointing to each other. Draw the arms to the sides, and lift the hands to the shoulder level, with the palms up. Straighten the arms with the fingertips of the two hands pointing front left and front right, respectively. Stretch the upper body upwards, and turn the head left. Turn the palms down, and lower the arms slowly to the sides. Repeat 15 times. Finally, click the teeth, gargle with the saliva and swallow. Inhale and exhale as in the previous form.

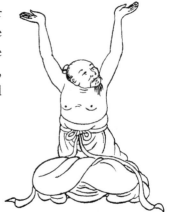

Figure 9.17
Seated Exercise at Cold Dew,
October

SEATED EXERCISE AT DESCENT OF FROST, OCTOBER

Application: Rheumatism and numbness in the waist and legs, inability to bend the hip joint, tearing pain in the calves, aching neck, back, waist and buttocks, bulge in the navel, muscular atrophy, stool with pus and blood, distended lower abdomen, difficulty in urination, chronic piles and rectocele.

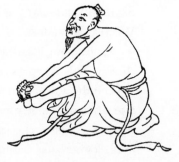

Figure 9.18
Seated Exercise at Descent of
Frost, October

Steps: Every morning between 1 am and 5 am sit with the legs stretched forward. Hold the soles of the feet with the corresponding hands, and bend the knees slightly. Push the feet forwards, and pull them back with the hands. Exert strength for a few seconds, and then bend the knees and arms. Repeat 35 times. Finally, click the teeth, gargle with the saliva and swallow. Inhale and exhale as in the previous form.

SEATED EXERCISE AT THE BEGINNING OF WINTER, NOVEMBER

Application: Stagnant harmful factors in the chest and flanks, physical weakness, inability to bend the waist due to pain, dry throat, pale face, distended chest, vomiting and hiccupping, headache, swollen cheeks, inflamed eyes, pain in the lower flanks tearing the lower abdomen, and distended limbs.

Steps: Every morning between 1 am and 5 am sit cross-legged. Lift the hands along the sides to the front of the chest with the palms up, and draw the forearms to the sides. Push the palms forward, and turn the head to the left. Then lower the arms slowly, and turn the face to the front. Repeat the arm movements, and turn the head to the right. Repeat 15 times on each side. Finally, click the teeth, gargle with the saliva and swallow. Inhale and exhale as in the previous form.

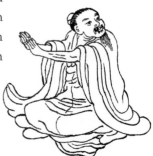

Figure 9.19
Seated Exercise at the Beginning
of Winter, November

Seated Exercise at Slight Snow, November

Application: Rheumatism and heat in the wrists and elbows, painful lower abdomen (women), hernia, enuresis and swollen testes (men), spasm, shrinking genitals, diarrhea due to deficiency in the kidneys, asthma, coughing and panic.

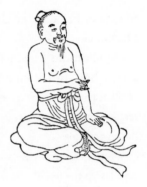

Figure 9.20
Seated Exercise at Slight
Snow, November

Steps: Every morning between 1 am and 5 am sit cross-legged. Press the left hand on the left knee, with the fingertips pointing forward. Pull the left elbow to the right with the right hand while the left elbow tries to pull to the left. Keep the tension for a few seconds. Repeat 15 times on each side. Finally, click the teeth, gargle with the saliva and swallow. Inhale and exhale as in the previous form.

Standing Exercise at Great Snow, December

Application: Rheumatism in the feet and knees, heat in the mouth and dry tongue, swollen throat, blockage of *qi* in the lungs and respiratory tract, irritation, heart pains and damp genitals.

Steps: Every day between 11 pm and 3 am stand with the feet shoulder-width apart and the knees slightly bent. Stretch the arms on both sides in line with the shoulders, with the palms erect. March on the spot. After a while click the teeth, gargle with the saliva and swallow. Inhale and exhale as in the previous form.

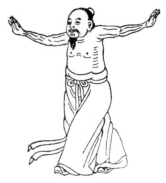

Figure 9.21
Standing Exercise at Great
Snow, December

Seated Exercise at Winter Solstice, December

Application: Chill and dampness in the hands and feet meridians, pain in the backbone and thighs, flaccid feet, somnolence, hot and painful soles of the feet, aching navel and flanks, distended chest, pain in the abdomen, constipation, swollen neck, coughing and coldness in the waist.

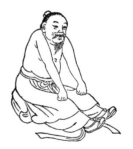

Figure 9.22
Seated Exercise at Winter
Solstice, December

Steps: Every day between 11 pm and 3 am sit with the legs stretched forward and shoulder-width apart. Press the hollow fists on the knees with the elbows pointing front left and front right, respectively, and the thumb sides of the fists toward the abdomen. Bend the upper body forward, and press the fists hard against the knees. Then shift the center of gravity back, and press the fists gently on the knees. Repeat 15 times. Finally, click the teeth, gargle with the saliva and swallow. Inhale and exhale as in the previous form.

SEATED EXERCISE AT SLIGHT COLD, JANUARY

Application: Stagnant *qi*, vomiting soon after eating, stomachache, distended abdomen, fatigue and weakness, acute heart pain, constipation, difficulty in urination, and jaundice.

Steps: Every day between 11 pm and 3 am sit cross-legged. Place the right thigh on the left calf, and press the left palm on the inside of the sole of the right foot. Stretch up the right hand with the palm up and fingertips pointing right, as if holding up the sky. Turn the head to look

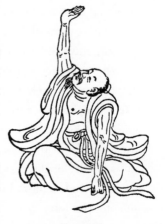

Figure 9.23
Seated Exercise at Slight Cold, January

at the right hand. Then switch the positions of the hands and feet. Repeat 15 times on each side. Finally, click the teeth, gargle with the saliva and swallow. Inhale and exhale as in the previous form.

SEATED EXERCISE AT GREAT COLD, JANUARY

Application: Harmful stagnant factors in the meridians, painful root of the tongue, paralysis or inability to lie down, swollen thighs and knees, pain in the feet, distended abdomen and rumbling stomach, diarrhea, and swollen feet.

Steps: Every day between 11 pm and 3 am sit with the left hip on the left heel, and stretch the right leg forward. Prop the right heel on the ground, and bend the upper body backwards. Prop the arms on the ground behind on the left and right respectively, with the fingertips facing left and right respectively. Shift the center of gravity backwards and then forwards. Switch the positions of the legs, and repeat 15 times on each side. Finally, click the teeth, gargle with the saliva and swallow. Inhale and exhale as in the previous form.

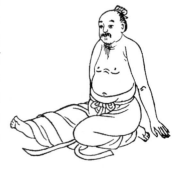

Figure 9.24
Seated Exercise at Great
Cold, January

X

CHEN XIYI'S SLEEPING EXERCISES

Chen Xiyi's Sleeping Exercises, recorded in the *Eight Essays on Health Preservation*, are said to have been created by Taoist priest Chen Tuan of the early Song Dynasty.

After failing the highest imperial examinations, Chen Tuan (?-989) became a hermit on Mount Wudang. It is said that he exercised a firm diet and abstained from grain while drinking several cups of wine every day during his over 20 years of seclusion. Later he moved to Mount Hua. Chen Tuan was very fond of reading *The Book of Changes* (*Yi Jing*). Song Emperor Taizong (reigned 976-997) lavished gifts on Chen Tuan, and granted him the title Xiyi Xiansheng (Gentleman Who Sees and Hears Nothing). Chen Tuan's works include the *Chart of the Infinite* and the *Chart of Anterior Heaven*. Legend has it that he often lay on a rock to do exercises on Mount Hua. His way of exercising was called "Chen Xiyi's Sleeping Exercises" by later generations.

The following illustrations are based on those for Chen Xiyi's Sleeping Exercises drawn by a contemporary, Zhang Tingdong.

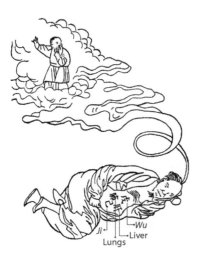

Figure 10.1
Sleeping Exercise on the Left Side

Ji, the sixth of the Ten Heavenly Stems

Wu, the fifth of the Ten Heavenly Stems

Lie on the left side, with the left elbow bent. Rest the head on the left palm, with the left ear between the parted thumb and index finger. Straighten the back slightly. Bend the left knee so that the left thigh touches the lower abdomen. Place the right leg on the left one in the same position, and cover the navel with the right palm. Imagine the breath going down to the navel, and coordinate the mind with the breathing. Gradually forget all external things, and enter into a state of deep meditation.

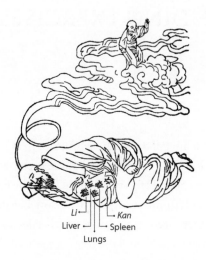

Figure 10.2
Sleeping Exercise on the Right Side

Lie on the right side. The other requirements
are the same as for the previous exercise.

XI

Eight-section Brocade Standing Exercises

Eight-section Brocade is a set of dynamic exercises for health preservation composed of eight parts. It is recorded that these exercises appeared at the end of the Northern Song Dynasty (960–1127). In the early Southern Song Dynasty (1127–1279) an anonymous person began to edit the materials describing Eight-section Brocade, which later developed into two schools—the northern school and the southern school. The northern school, also known as the martial school, features strength and the horse stance; the southern school, also known as the civil school, is characterized by suppleness and an upright stance, and so these were also called the Eight-section Brocade Standing Exercises.

Both the forms and contents of the Eight-section Brocade Standing Exercises underwent certain changes as time went by. In the latter half of the 19th century the exercises were practiced as follows: "Upholding the sky to recuperate the *sanjiao*; drawing a bow on both sides as if shooting an eagle; raising a single arm to regulate the spleen and stomach; turning the head to cure feebleness and internal damage; shaking the head and swaying the hips to remove internal heat; bumping seven times to dispel all diseases; clenching the fist with wide-open glaring eyes to increase strength; clasping the feet with the hands to solidify the kidneys and waist." Volume 16 of *An Illustrated Book of Exercises to Benefit the Internal Organs–Promoting the Metabolism, Limbering Up the Tendons and Refreshing the Marrow* compiled by Zhou Shuguan in 1895 provides illustrations and introductions for this version, and points out that the Eight-section Brocade Standing Exercises focus on stimulating circulation of the blood and *qi*. The following is reprinted according to the 1930 lithographic version of the book.

HOLDING THE SKY UP TO RECUPERATE THE SANJIAO

Application: Tight chest, distended abdomen and poor appetite caused by diseases in the *sanjiao*, lungs and spleen.

Steps: Stand splayfooted with naturally straight legs. Relax the hips and lower the waist. Draw the chest inward, and hunch the back slightly, making the armpits hollow. Draw the chin slightly inward, and let the neck droop while pulling the head up. Look straight ahead without concentration, and let the arms hang loosely at the sides with the fingers naturally bent. Relax the shoulders, and take slow, long, even and deep breaths.

After finishing the above preparations, start practicing the exercise as follows: draw the hands to the front of the abdomen. Straighten and clasp the fingers with the fingertips of one hand pointing to those of the other and the palms up. Raise the hands to the front of the chest. Continue to lift the arms while rotating the palms, and finally stretch the arms upwards with the palms up, as if holding the sky up. During the whole process from the preparations to the final position, keep the mouth closed and rest the tip of the tongue on the palate. Inhale through the nose in a slow, long, even and deep breath. Pause for one or two seconds in the position of holding up the sky. Part the arms gradually, and lower them to the sides while exhaling through the mouth in a slow, long, even and deep breath. Repeat the whole process seven times. Keep your eyes fixed on the hands. (Figure 11.1)

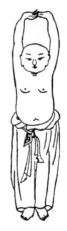

Figure 11.1
Holding the Sky Up to
Recuperate the *Sanjiao*

SHOOTING AN ARROW AT AN EAGLE

Application: Auxiliary treatment for lung diseases, and pains in the shoulders and arms, and as rehabilitation in the case of lung diseases.

Steps: Stand with feet apart at shoulder width and arms hanging at the sides. Face the front. Raise the arms slowly leftward, with the thumb sides of the hollow fists upward, till the left hand is in line with the left shoulder. Stretch the left hand in this direction, and raise the index finger while bending the right elbow and pulling it toward the rear right with the right hand in front of the right shoulder. Squat and pause for one or two seconds. Then straighten the legs, and return the arms to the beginning position along the original route. Repeat seven times on each side. Inhale at the very beginning of each repetition, and pause for a while at the position of drawing a bow. Then exhale slowly as the arms descend. Shift the eyes with the movement of the hands, and look into the distance at the pauses. (Figure 11.2)

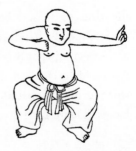

Figure 11.2
Shooting an Arrow at
an Eagle

RAISING AN ARM TO REGULATE THE SPLEEN AND STOMACH

Application: Upset spleen and stomach, diseases caused by stagnant and disordered flow of *qi*, numbness, and pains in the shoulders and back.

Steps: Do the preparations as in the previous form. Draw the hands to the front of the lower abdomen, with the palms up and the fingertips of one hand pointing to those of the other. Raise the hands to a point between the chest and abdomen. Turn the left palm down, and press it downward behind the buttocks. Meanwhile, turn the right palm inward, downward and outward, and then lift it up. Align the fingertips of both hands vertically at a distance from each other. Straighten the arms, and pause for a while. Then turn the palms, and draw the hands to a spot midway between the chest and abdomen, with the palms opposite each other. Repeat seven times on each side. Finally, draw the hands to the spot between the chest and abdomen, with both palms down. Press the hands down, and return to the starting position. Inhale at the beginning of this exercise, and hold the breath when holding one arm on high. Then exhale slowly as the arms descend, and hold the breath when turning the palms. Shift the eyes with the upward movement of the hands. (Figure 11.3)

TURNING THE HEAD TO CURE FEEBLENESS AND INTERNAL DAMAGE

Application: Various kinds of feebleness and internal damage.

Steps: Do the preparations as in the previous form. Stand naturally, with the arms hanging at the sides. Turn the upper body and head slowly leftwards as far as possible, and pause for one or two seconds. Then turn the upper body and head slowly rightwards as far as possible. Repeat seven times on each side. Start inhaling at the beginning of this exercise, taking in the maximum breath when turned to the extreme side. Exhale when starting turning to the front, and breathe out as deeply as possible. Keep looking straight ahead as the upper body and head turn. (Figure 11.4)

SHAKING THE HEAD AND SWAYING THE HIPS TO REMOVE INTERNAL HEAT

Application: Excessive internal heat, stress, dark-red urine, and pains in the shoulders, waist and legs.

Steps: Stand with the feet apart at shoulder width, with the arms hanging naturally at the sides and the eyes looking straight ahead. Bend forward at the waist and half-squat, with the hands placed on the knees.

Turn the upper body and head towards the front left while lifting the upper body slightly and raising the head. Sway the bottom toward rear right. Then bow the head, stoop toward the front left, and sway the upper body to the front right. Lift the upper body slightly, raising the head at the same time. Repeat the movements seven times on each side. Inhale slowly when turning from front to front left or front right, and pause for a while. Exhale in the opposite direction. Shift the eyes with the movement of the upper body. (Figure 11.5)

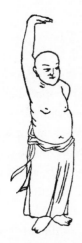

Figure 11.3
Raising an Arm to Regulate
the Spleen and Stomach

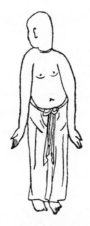

Figure 11.4
Turning the Head to Cure
Feebleness and Internal
Damage

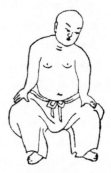

Figure 11.5
Shaking the Head and
Swaying the Hips to Remove
Internal Heat

Bumping Seven Times to Dispel All Diseases

Application: Diseases caused by disordered circulation of blood and *qi*, and discomfort or pain in the neck, nape, waist, knees, ankles and toes.

Steps: Relax the whole body, and let the arms hang naturally at the sides. The shoulders should be slightly shrugged. Lift the heels three to six cm off the ground, and then lower them rapidly, at the same time bending the knees slightly. Repeat the bumping movement seven times. Inhale when lifting the heels, and exhale when lowering them. Keep looking straight ahead. (Figure 11.6)

Clenching the Fists with Wide-open, Glaring Eyes to Increase Strength

Application: Depletion of *qi*, shortness of breath, fatigue, indigestion or lack of appetite, rheumatism, numbness and pains in the upper limbs.

Steps: Stand with the feet the length of one foot apart, with the arms half bent and the palms up. Clench the fists, and push them forward slowly. Turn the forearms inward at shoulder height, with the thumb sides of the fists opposite each other. Pause for one or two seconds, and then draw the fists back to the waist following the original route. With the fists still clenched, push them to each side respectively with the thumb sides forward. Hold the arms at shoulder height, and then draw the fists back to the waist. Repeat seven times in each direction. Exhale when pushing the fists out, and inhale when drawing them back to the waist. Practice the whole exercise with wide-open, glaring eyes. Look straight ahead when pushing the fists forward. Look once in each direction when pushing the fists out from the sides. (Figure 11.7)

Clasping the Feet with the Hands to Solidify the Kidneys and Waist

Application: Weak liver and kidneys, aching and feeble waist, back, chest and knees.

Steps: Stand with feet two fist-widths apart. Push both hands forwards, and then raise them upwards. Bend the upper body forward, and try to press the chest against the thighs. Stretch the arms downwards, with the hands touching the feet or clasping the toes. Pause for one or two seconds, and then lift the upper body and arms slowly. Repeat seven times. Exhale when bending forward, and inhale when straightening the back. Shift the eyes with the movements of the hands. (Figure 11.8)

Take a five-minute walk to conclude the Eight-section Brocade Standing Exercises.

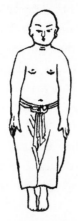

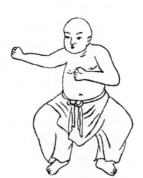

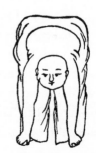

Figure 11.6
Bumping Seven Times to
Dispel All Diseases

Figure 11.7
Clenching the Fists with
Wide-open, Glaring Eyes to
Increase Strength

Figure 11.8
Clasping the Feet with the
Hands to Solidify the Kidneys
and Waist

XII

EIGHT-SECTION BROCADE SEATED EXERCISES

The Eight-section Brocade Seated Exercises developed from the southern school of Eight-section Brocade Exercises, which also include the Eight-section Brocade Standing Exercises. Volume 19 of the Taoist compilation *Ten Books on the Cultivation of Perfection (Xiuzhen Shishu)* of the Jin–Yuan period (13th–14th centuries) was the first book to depict the Eight-section Brocade Seated Exercises, with both illustrations and essays. Although the seated exercises underwent some changes, the basic patterns were set down in this book. *Illustrated Formulas for the Eight-section Brocade Seated and Standing Exercises*, compiled by physician Lou Jie of the Qing Dynasty in 1876 incorporated 18 forms of such sitting and standing exercises (see Chapter XXIII). The following illustrations are based on those in the *Illustrated Formulas for Eight-section Brocade Seated and Standing Exercises*.

SECTION ONE: CLICKING THE TEETH IN DEEP MEDITATION

Sit cross-legged, with the eyes closed and the fists clenched. Concentrate the mind, and meditate. Click the teeth 36 times. Put the hands behind the neck, and take nine silent breaths. Then cover the ears with the palms, and tap the back of the head 24 times each with the middle finger tucked under the index finger of each hand. (Figure 12.1)

SECTION TWO: SHAKING THE NAPE

Clasp the hands. Shake the head and shoulders around 24 times. (Figure 12.2)

SECTION THREE: GARGLING WITH THE SALIVA, AND SWALLOWING IT

Stir the tongue around the mouth 36 times to produce saliva. Gargle with the saliva 36 times to make a mouthful. Swallow it in three gulps as if forcing something hard down the throat. (Figure 12.3)

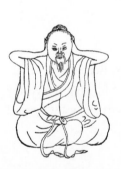

Figure 12.1
Section One: Clicking the
Teeth in Deep Meditation

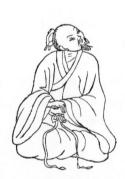

Figure 12.2
Section Two: Shaking
the Nape

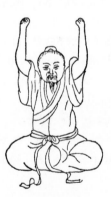

Figure 12.3
Section Three: Gargling with
the Saliva, and Swallowing it

Section Four: Massaging Shentang

Inhale deeply through the nose. After a while, rub the hands together until they are warm. Massage *shentang* with both hands 36 times. *Shentang*, i.e. *jingmen*, refers to the two softest areas in the lower back. Clench the fists, and inhale deeply. Imagine that a fire is spreading from the heart to *dantian*, until that area feels extremely hot. (Figure 12.4)

Section Five: Rotating one Arm like a Windlass

Bow the head and bend the elbows. Rotate the left shoulder and arm 36 times like a windlass. Then repeat on the right side. (Figure 12.5)

Section Six: Rotating Both Arms like Windlasses Simultaneously

Simultaneously rotate both arms like windlasses 36 times. Imagine that a fire is spreading from the *dantian* to the head. Inhale deeply through the nose, and then stretch the crossed legs forward. (Figure 12.6)

Section Seven: Holding up the Sky and Pressing upon the Vertex

Sit cross-legged with the fingers interlaced. Stretch the hands up as if holding up the sky, and then press upon the vertex. Repeat nine times. Exert the full strength when raising the hands as if holding something extremely heavy. At the same time, pull the upper body and waist upward to the utmost. (Figure 12.7)

SECTION EIGHT: BENDING FORWARD AND CLASPING THE FEET

Stretch the hands forward to clasp the arches of the feet 20 times. Then sit cross-legged with the fists clenched. Gather a mouthful of saliva. Gargle with it and then swallow it. Repeat the whole process 24 times. Imagine that a fire from the *dantian* spreads upwards over the body. Sit still for a while. (Figure 12.8)

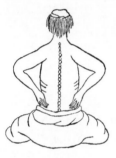

Figure 12.4
Section Four: Massaging
Shentang

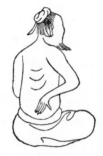

Figure 12.5
Section Five: Rotating one
Arm like a Windlass

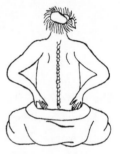

Figure 12.6
Section Six: Rotating Both
Arms like Windlasses
Simultaneously

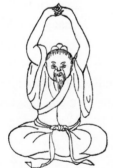

Figure 12.7
Section Seven: Holding up
the Sky and Pressing upon
the Vertex

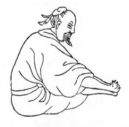

Figure 12.8
Section Eight: Bending
Forward and Clasping
the Feet

XIII

Twelve-section Brocade Exercises

The patterns of Twelve-section Brocade Exercises, derived from the Eight-section Brocade Exercises, were basically finalized in the early Ming Dynasty. The formulas in verse of the *Twelve-section Brocade Exercises included in the Illustrated Exercises for Prolonging Life* (*Shoushi Chuanzhen*) by Xu Wenbi of the Qing Dynasty were the same as those of the Eight-section Brocade Exercises in the *daoyin* methods incorporated in the *Essentials for Gaining Longevity* (*Xiuling Yaozhi*) by Leng Qian, *Eight Essays on Health Preservation* (*Zunsheng Bajian*) by Gao Lian, and *Major Mottos for Health Preservation* (*Leixiu Yaojue*) by Hu Wenhuan, of the Ming Dynasty, except for a few characters. The expositions on the methods of practicing the exercises in those books vary only in length. The following illustrations are based on those of the block-printed edition of the *Illustrated Exercises for Prolonging Life*.

Sitting in Meditation with the Eyes Closed and Fists Clenched

Sit cross-legged with the eyes closed, and concentrate the mind. Straighten the back and waist without leaning on anything. Clenching the fists can dispel any distracting thoughts. Sit still in deep meditation to visualize the spirit. (Figure 13.1)

Clicking the Teeth 36 Times and Embracing the Head

Click the teeth 36 times to concentrate the spirit inside the body. Embrace the back of the head with the fingers interlaced, and press the palms upon the *erhmen*, the grooves along the edge of the ears. Count silently while breathing nine times gently through the nose. (Figure 13.2)

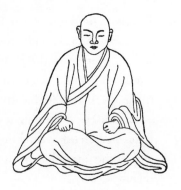

Figure 13.1
Sitting in Meditation with the Eyes Closed and Fists Clenched

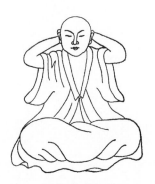

Figure 13.2
Clicking the Teeth 36 Times and Embracing the Head

95

PATTING THE BACK OF THE HEAD

Cover the ears with the palms. Press the index finger upon the middle finger of each hand and pat the back of the head firmly with the index finger slipping off the middle finger each time, as if tapping a drum. Repeat 24 times on each side. Lower the arms to the sides, and let them rest there with the fists clenched. (Figure 13.3)

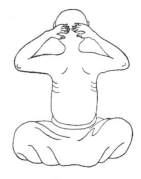

Figure 13.3
Patting the Back of the Head

SHAKING THE NAPE

Sit cross-legged, and bow the head. Shake the head and shoulders 24 times on each side. (Figure 13.4)

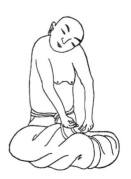

Figure 13.4
Shaking the Nape

GARGLING WITH THE SALIVA

Prop the tongue against the upper palate and stir it around the mouth to produce saliva. Gargle with the saliva 36 times, and swallow it noisily in three gulps. Imagine that the saliva is being sent down to the *dantian* with *qi* following it. (Figure 13.5)

HOLDING THE BREATH AND RUBBING THE HANDS

Breathe in through the nose, and then hold the breath. Rub the hands together until they feel hot. Then immediately massage the Jingmen, the two soft areas in the lower back, 36 times while exhaling through the nose. Lower the arms to the sides, and let them rest there with the fists clenched. (Figure 13.6)

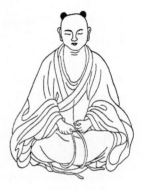

Figure 13.5
Gargling with the Saliva

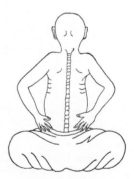

Figure 13.6
Holding the Breath and Rubbing the Hands

Holding the Breath and Imagining a Fire Burning at the Dantian

Hold the breath and imagine that a fire is spreading from the heart to the *dantian*. Breathe out slowly through the nose when a hot feeling ensues. (Figure 13.7)

Rotating the Arms Alternately

Bend the elbows, and rotate the left shoulder and arm 36 times like a windlass. Then repeat on the right side. (Figure 13.8)

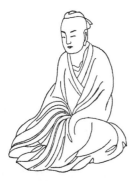

Figure 13.7
Holding the Breath and Imagining a
Fire Burning at the *Dantian*

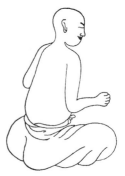

Figure 13.8
Rotating the Arms Alternately

STRETCHING THE LEGS AND RAISING THE INTERLOCKED HANDS

Stretch the crossed legs forward, and interlace the fingers. Place the backs of the hands upon the vertex, and then raise the arms with the palms up, as if holding a heavy stone. At the same time, pull the upper body upward, and pause for a while. Replace the hands on the vertex, and stretch them upwards again after a short pause. Repeat nine times. (Figure 13.9)

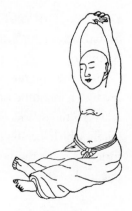

Figure 13.9
Stretching the Legs and Raising
the Interlocked Hands

PULLING THE SOLES AND BOWING THE HEAD

Unlock the fingers, and clasp the soles of the feet with the hands. Bow the head low as you pull on the soles. Repeat 12 times. Finally, draw back the hands, and sit cross-legged with the fists clenched. (Figure 13.10)

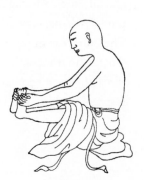

Figure 13.10
Pulling the Soles and Bowing
the Head

Gargling with the Saliva and Swallowing it in Three Gulps for Three Rounds

Stir the tongue around the mouth to produce a mouthful of saliva. Gargle with the saliva 36 times, and swallow it in three gulps loudly, which is counted as one round. Do this thrice to make the body's meridians regular. (Figure 13.11)

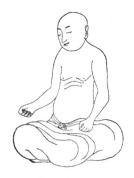

Figure 13.11
Gargling with the Saliva and Swallowing it in Three Gulps for Three Rounds

Transferring Qi from the Kidneys

Imagine fiery *qi* at the *dantian*, and hold the breath as if suppressing defecation. Concentrate and direct the *qi* to the anus, and then up to the waist, back, nape, back of the head and vertex. Then direct *qi* from the forehead down to the temples, in front of the root of the ears, cheeks, throat, heart and the *dantian*. Imagine that a fire is spreading throughout the body. (Figure 13.12)

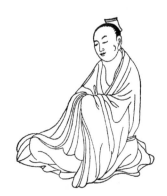

Figure 13.12
Transferring *Qi* from the Kidneys

XIV

Xiaoyao Zi *Daoyin* Method

The following descriptions of the Xiaoyao Zi *Daoyin* Method are based on the records in a monograph on *qigong–Xiaoyao Zi Daoyin Formulas*, of which the name of the author and the date of composition are both unknown. The *Essentials for Gaining Longevity (Xiuling Yaozhi)* by Leng Qian of the early Ming Dynasty referred to it as "*daoyin* formulas in verse." In 1548 Hu Wenhuan incorporated it into the *Major Mottos for Health Preservation (Leixiu Yaojue)*, and renamed it "Xiaoyao Zi *Daoyin* Formulas." Both books included 16 lines of five-character verse, of which 15 lines were accompanied by illustrations by the end of the Qing Dynasty, with the line "Light food serves as a tonic" as the exception. The illustrations are reproduced from the Qing Dynasty 1911 handwritten copy of the *Formulas of Seated Exercises for Preventing Diseases*.

Swallowing the Saliva Saves Future Trouble

Sit upright immediately after waking up, and concentrate the mind. Place the tongue against the upper palate. Close the mouth and regulate the breathing to produce a mouthful of saliva. Swallow it in three gulps and imagine sending it down. Constant practice prevents diseases in the internal organs and ensures the smooth flow of blood and *qi* in the limbs. This exercise wards off all diseases, and leads to longevity. (Figure 14.1)

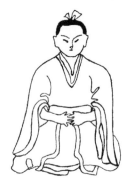

Figure 14.1
Swallowing the Saliva Saves
Future Trouble

Fire Leads to Lifelong Health

Between midnight and noon, sit on the heels, and place the hands on the ground behind. Close the eyes slightly, and imagine a fire starting at the Yongquan point at the center of the sole of the left foot and going up to the left side of the waist through the left leg, the inward side of the left shoulder blade, the external occipital protuberance and vertex; then downwards to the left cheek, left collar bone, left nipple and the *dantian*. Repeat this circulation

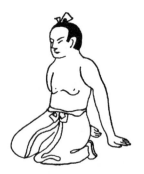

Figure 14.2
Fire Leads to Lifelong Health

three times on each side. Constant practice guarantees smooth flow in all meridians, gets rid of stagnation in the internal organs, and regulates the limbs and all the bones. (Figure 14.2)

A HEALTHY MENTALITY AVERTS
NOCTURNAL EMISSIONS

A feeling of intense heat inside the body and mental fatigue when attempting to move can result in nocturnal emission. Before going to sleep, lie on the back. Regulate the breath, and concentrate the mind, with the eyes slightly closed. Rub the navel with the left hand 14 times, and repeat with the right hand. Rub the left flank with the left hand up and down 14 times, and repeat with the right hand. Then sit up, and press the hands on the Shenyu point on each side of the lower back. Shake the upper body left and right seven times each. Take a deep breath, and send it to the *dantian*. Clench the fists for 15 minutes. Finally, lie down on the side with bent knees. (Figure 14.3)

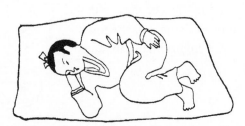

Figure 14.3
A Healthy Mentality Averts Nocturnal Emissions

CONCENTRATION AND MEDITATION SOLIDIFIES THE DANTIAN

Entanglement in all kinds of worries and problems tires the body and consumes energy. One who knows how to preserve health always concentrates the mind and circulates *qi* quietly in daily life to strengthen the *dantian*, and thus maintains vitality and prolongs life. (Figure 14.4)

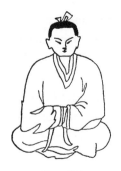

Figure 14.4
Concentration and Meditation
Strengthens the *Dantian*

EXHALING REMOVES INDIGESTION AND DEPRESSION

Frequent indigestion and depression harm the spleen and stomach, ailments which are difficult to cure by medicine. It is advisable to avoid gluttony and anger. Once indigestion or depression occurs, sit upright and raise the arms, with the fingers interlaced. Raise the shoulders and upper body. Lower the arms to the sides, hold the breath and fill the abdomen with *qi*. Exhale slowly through the mouth. Repeat 35 times to relieve the stomach and abdomen. (Figure 14.5)

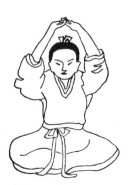

Figure 14.5
Exhaling Dispels Indigestion
and Depression

Cupping the External Genitalia Dispels Cold

Deficiency of vital *qi* and slack muscles invite cold and gloom. Sit cross-legged, and cup the external genitalia with both hands. Close the mouth, and hold the breath. Imagine vital *qi* rising from the sacrum, through the Jiaji points along both sides of the spine, to the head and expelling the harmful factors. Then bow the head, and bend the upper body until sweat forms. Cold will then be dispelled. (Figure 14.6)

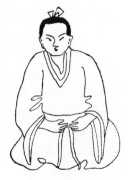

Figure 14.6
Cupping the External
Genitalia Dispels Cold

Clicking the Teeth Prevents Dental Diseases

Dental diseases are caused by excessive heat in the spleen and stomach. After waking in the early morning, click the teeth 36 times. Lick the gums with the tongue to produce a mouthful of saliva, and swallow it. Repeat three times. Clench the teeth during urination, and release the tension after finishing. Constant practice of these exercises prevents dental diseases. (Figure 14.7)

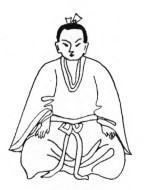

Figure 14.7
Clicking the Teeth Prevents
Dental Diseases

Looking up Averts Gray Hairs

Too much thinking wearies the mind, causes depletion of *qi* and blood, and results in gray hairs. At midnight or in the morning, sit cross-legged, with the hands clasped. Concentrate the mind, and stare up towards the forehead with shining eyes. Meanwhile, imagine that *qi* and blood from the sacrum are going up through Mingmen, known as the gate of vitality (area between the kidneys), Jiaji, Yuzhen (at the lower rear part of the head) and Baihui (on the top of the head), and then going down through the Yintang point (midway between the eyebrows), Shanzhong (midway between the nipples) and navel to the lower abdomen. Repeat this circulation nine times. Constant practice brings abundant energy, *qi* and blood, and wards off the graying of hair. (Figure 14.8)

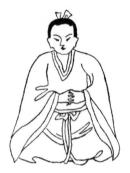

Figure 14.8
Looking up Averts Gray Hair

Turning the Eyeballs Clears Mist

Excessive heat and depletion of *qi*, and weak liver and kidneys result in mist in the eyes, which will deteriorate into blindness if left untreated for a long time. After waking up early in the morning, sit cross-legged, with the mouth closed. Half-close the eyes, leaving a small gap between the eyelids. Turn both eyeballs around at the same time, looking left, up, right and down, and then turn them in the other direction. Repeat seven times in each direction. Close the eyes tightly for a while and suddenly open the eyes wide. Constant practice clears away mist from the eyes. It is also advisable to abstain from sex and reading small print. (Figure 14.9)

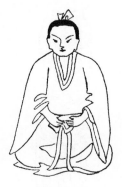

Figure 14.9
Turning the Eyeballs
Clears Mist

Covering the Ears Removes Giddiness

Wind and excessive internal heat cause headaches of various types, including migraine, and can lead to wind stroke and aphasia. Sit upright, and cover the ears with the palms, with the thumbs down and fingers pointing backwards. Move the head forwards, backwards, left and right, seven times in each direction. Imagine that vital *qi* is rushing from the lower abdomen to the top of the head. Constant practice dispels wind and refreshes the mind. (Figure 14.10)

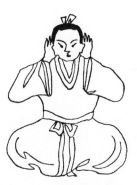

Figure 14.10
Covering the Ears Removes
Giddiness

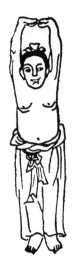

Figure 14.11
Holding the Hands Up
Invigorates the Limbs

Holding the Hands Up Invigorates the Limbs

An old Chinese saying goes: "A door-hinge is never worm-eaten." The limbs need regular exercise. Imitating a bear climbing and a bird spreading its wings, breathing in and out, and *daoyin* exercises are all conducive to preserving health. Stand straight with the palms up and the fingers of one hand pointing to those of the other. Raise the hands to the lower abdomen, navel, upper abdomen and front of the chest. Rotate the forearms and palms inward, and stretch the hands up with the palms up, as if holding a heavy stone. Meanwhile, march in place seven times with each foot, bringing the knees up as high as possible. Retrace the original route with the hands, and exhale three times through the mouth. Repeat the whole exercise seven times. Constant practice limbers up the body and warms the feet. (Figure 14.11)

Face Massage Brings a Bright Look

A gaunt look implies too much thinking and laboring. After waking up early every morning, sit still with the eyes closed in deep meditation. Imagine that *qi* originating from the *dantian* is

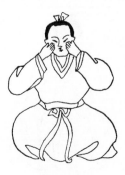

Figure 14.12
Face Massage Brings a
Bright Look

spreading throughout the body like ripples, from inside to outside. When a warm feeling is perceived rub the hands together till they are hot. Massage outward from the sides of the nose and from the middle of the forehead to the two sides seven times, respectively. Rub the face several times with saliva. Half a month of this practice will bring about a lustrously smooth skin. (Figure 14.12)

MASSAGE WHILE MEDITATING DISPELS STAGNANCY

Stagnant *qi* leads to pain, and stagnant blood results in swelling. To combat these conditions sit still in deep meditation, and focus the mind on the affected part. Massage the part with the thenar eminence of the left palm up and down seven times, first gently over a large area, gradually increasing the strength and reducing the area. Repeat the whole process seven times with each hand. Then apply saliva to the affected part. Consecutive practice for seven days both morning and evening will dispel stagnancy and smooth the flow of blood and *qi*. (Figure 14.13)

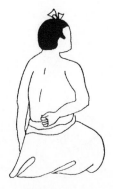

Figure 14.13
Massage while Meditating
Dispels Stagnancy

Embracing the Lower Abdomen Solidifies the Dantian

Sit still, and place the hands on the lower abdomen. Imagine that the vital *qi* enters the *dantian*, and then spirals clockwise and counterclockwise three times each. One hundred days of practice solidifies the *dantian* and enriches vital *qi*. Avoid heavy labor during the practice period. (Figure 14.14)

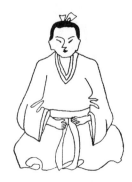

Figure 14.14
Embracing the Lower Abdomen
Solidifies the *Dantian*

Broad-mindedness Contributes to Health

Temper the character and be broad-minded about gains and losses, and fame and power. A constant happy mood contributes to health. (Figure 14.15)

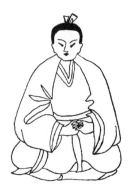

Figure 14.15
Broad-mindedness
Contributes to Health

XV

VARIOUS *DAOYIN* EXERCISES OF THE IMMORTALS

The illustrations for the Various *Daoyin* Exercises of the Immortals are based on those for *Forty-nine Prescriptions Left by Immortals* by Luo Hongxian of the Ming Dynasty.

Luo Hongxian became the Number One Scholar, a title conferred on the person who came first in the highest imperial examination, in 1529. Luo Hongxian had been fond of health-preserving exercises since he was young. During a visit to Luoyang in 1561 he met an immortal whose surname was Zhu in the Lichun Garden. Zhu gave Luo a book named *Real Rhyme of Hygiene*. Luo perused the book, and found that it recorded all kinds of formulas and prescriptions concocted by ancient immortals for directing qi. Luo found them effective after trying them. He edited the book into two volumes, titled *Forty-nine Prescriptions Left by Immortals*. This book has been handed down to the present day. The first volume includes Knacks for Directing *Qi*, Key Principles for *Daoyin* and various immortals' methods of making internal and external elixirs. The second volume contains 49 prescriptions, each with title, illustration, application, steps, recipe and related poems. The *Forty-nine Prescriptions Left by Immortals* embraces both text and illustrations, both exercises and recipes. It was rare for old medical books to combine *qigong* with herbal recipes.

Various *Daoyin* Exercises of Immortals were incorporated into another book by Luo Hongxian, titled *Immortals' Methods of Longevity*. An enlarged edition of this book, compiled by Cao Ruoshui of the Qing Dynasty, consisting of four volumes, is extant. The first volume collects Taoist secrets of preserving health. The second volume focuses on *daoyin* exercises, including the Eight-section Brocade Seated Exercises and Twenty-four-Seasonal-Division-Points Seated Exercises. The third introduces various *daoyin* exercises of the immortals, and the fourth explains the essentials for prolonging life. The block-printed edition of Cao Ruoshui's enlarged version, published in 1832, incorporated only 42 illustrations for the various *daoyin* exercises of the immortals, and the following illustrations are based on these. The seven missing ones—Qiu Changchun Turning the Well-pulley, Ma Danyang Reaching the Fire Phases of Cosmic Orbit, Zhang Ziyang Lifting a Millstone, Huang Huagu Lying on Her Side, Zhang Wumeng Standing on One Foot, Xia Yunfeng Bending over the Ground and Hao Taigu Upholding the Sky—are based on a Qing transcript of *Forty-nine Prescriptions Left by Immortals*. Two sections of texts, recipes and poems have been omitted. The names mentioned in the captions of illustrations are all immortals in ancient Chinese mythology.

Li Laojun Playing the Zither

Application: Prolonged yellow complexion and edema.

Steps: Sit cross-legged and rub the palms against the knees. Meditate in silence until *qi* circulates throughout the body. Then take 49 breaths, and direct *qi* throughout the body. In this way, *qi* and blood can circulate through the body smoothly, and illness will be eradicated. (Figure 15.1)

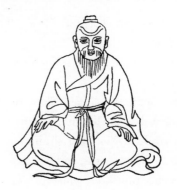

Figure 15.1
Li Laojun Playing the Zither

True Posture of Taiqing

Application: Abdominal pain and alternate heat and cold.

Steps: Sit upright, and embrace the lower abdomen with both hands. Focus the mind on the *dantian* until it becomes warm. Then take 49 breaths, and direct *qi* throughout the body. (Figure 15.2)

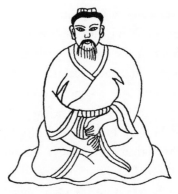

Figure 15.2
True Posture of Taiqing

Xu Shenweng Holding the Breath

Application: Distended stomach and abdomen.

Steps: Sit cross-legged. Place the right hand on the left shoulder and left hand on the right shoulder. Take 20 deep breaths, and direct *qi* throughout the body while turning the eyes to the left. Then repeat the process by turning the eyes to the right. (Figure 15.3)

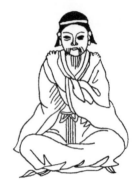

Figure 15.3
Xu Shenweng Holding the Breath

Li Tieguai Pointing Out the Road

Application: Paralysis.

Steps: Stand with the left foot in front of the right. Stretch out the right arm rightwards, and point the fingers in the same direction. Turn the head and eyes leftwards. Take 24 deep breaths, and direct *qi* throughout the body. Then put the right foot in front of the left, and repeat on the other side. (Figure 15.4)

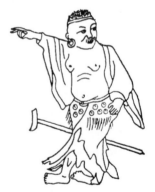

Figure 15.4
Li Tieguai Pointing Out the Road

He Xiangu Ascending to Heaven

Application: Dry cholera and abdominal pain.

Steps: Sit, clasping the knees with the hands and with the knees breast high. Kick the feet forward alternately nine times, and pull the knees backward nine times while taking 24 deep breaths and directing *qi* throughout the body. (Figure 15.5)

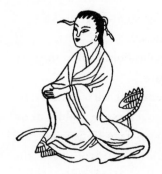

Figure 15.5
He Xiangu Ascending to Heaven

Bai Yuchan Mimicking a Tiger Pouncing on its Prey

Application: Dry cholera.

Steps: Lie on the stomach, and stretch the limbs upward as far as possible. Take 12 deep breaths, and direct *qi* throughout the body while waving the limbs left and right 15 times alternately. Then sit up naturally, and calm the breath. Take 14 deep breaths, and direct *qi* to the painful area. (Figure 15.6)

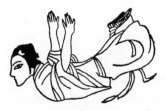

Figure 15.6
Bai Yuchan Mimicking a Tiger Pouncing on its Prey

Qiu Changchun Turning a Well-pulley

Application: Pain in the back and arms.

Steps: Sit on a chair, feet splayed. Press the palms upon the knees. Take 12 deep breaths, and direct *qi* throughout the body. Repeat 15 times a day. (Figure 15.7)

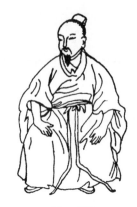

Figure 15.7
Qiu Changchun Turning a Well-pulley

Ma Danyang Conducting Full Circulation of Heat

Application: Depletion of vital energy.

Steps: Sit cross-legged, and rub the palms together until they are warm. Close the eyes lightly, and rub them with the palms. Then place the palms on the abdomen just below the ribs. Direct *qi* into the abdomen, and concentrate the mind at the *dantian*. Take 12 breaths, and direct *qi* throughout the body. (Figure 15.8)

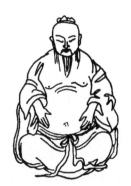

Figure 15.8
Ma Danyang Conducting Full Circulation of Heat

Zhang Ziyang Lifting a Millstone

Application: Distension and rumbling in the abdomen, and pain all over.

Steps: Stand with hands raised as if holding up the sky and feet firmly planted on the ground. Contract the anus while taking nine deep breaths, and direct *qi* throughout the body. (Figure 15.9)

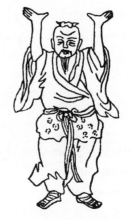

Figure 15.9
Zhang Ziyang Lifting a Millstone

Huang Huagu Lying on Her Side

Application: Fatigue and exhaustion.

Steps: Lie on the left side, left leg under the right. Bend the left leg slightly, and keep the right one straight. Put the left palm under the head. Clench the right fist, and place it on the right thigh. Take a deep breath, and concentrate the mind at the *dantian*. Then take 12 breaths, and direct *qi* throughout the body. (Figure 15.10)

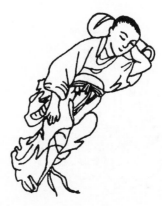

Figure 15.10
Huang Huagu Lying on Her Side

Han Zhongli Striking the Heavenly Drum

Application: Dizziness and grinding the teeth while sleeping.

Steps: Sit upright, cross-legged, and hold the breath. Cover the ears with the palms. Cross the index fingers over the middle fingers and flip the occiput with the index fingers as if striking a drum. Then click the teeth 36 times. (Figure 15.11)

Zhao Shangzao Stops Wet Dreams by Pulling and Rubbing the Feet

Application: Nocturnal emission.

Steps: Sit and pull the soles of the feet with hands. Pull the left sole with the left hand, and rub it with the right hand till it is hot. Take nine deep breaths, and direct *qi* throughout the body. Then change to the right side, and repeat the breathing and direction of *qi*. (Figure 15.12)

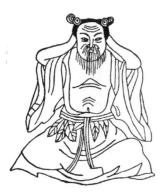

Figure 15.11
Han Zhongli Striking the Heavenly Drum

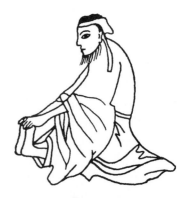

Figure 15.12
Zhao Shangzao Stops Wet Dreams by Pulling
and Rubbing the Feet

CELESTIAL MASTER XUJING'S SLEEPING METHOD

Application: Wet dreams.

Steps: Lie on the right side, right leg under the left. Bend the right leg and keep the right one straight. Place the right palm under the head, and hold the genitals with the left hand. Concentrate the mind, and meditate. Take 24 deep breaths, and direct *qi* throughout the body. (Figure 15.13)

LI QICHAN DISPERSING SEMEN

Application: Spermatorrhea, awake or asleep.

Steps: Sit up and rub the soles of the feet till they are warm. Take 30 deep breaths while rubbing each sole and direct *qi* throughout the body. (Figure 15.14)

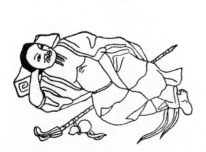

Figure 15.13
Celestial Master Xujing's Sleeping Method

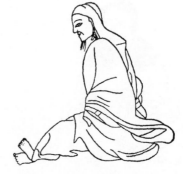

Figure 15.14
Li Qichan Dispersing Semen

Zhang Zhennu Concentrating the Mind

Application: Heart deficiency and pain.

Steps: Sit up, cross-legged, and press the palms upon the knees. Concentrate the mind at the *dantian*. Turn the eyes right, and direct *qi* upwards along the left side. Take 12 deep breaths. Then turn the eyes to the left, and direct *qi* upwards along the right side. Take another 12 deep breaths, and direct *qi* throughout the body. (Figure 15.15)

Wei Boyang Curing Paralysis

Application: Prolonged paralysis.

Steps: Sit up, cross-legged. Clench the left fist, and place it on the left side of the chest. Press the right palm on the right knee. Meditate, and direct *qi* throughout the body. Take six deep breaths. Repeat the whole process on the other side. (Figure 15.16)

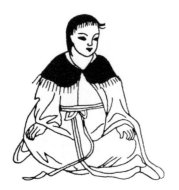

Figure 15.15
Zhang Zhennu Concentrating the Mind

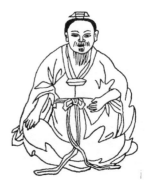

Figure 15.16
Wei Boyang Curing Paralysis

XUE DAOGUANG RUBBING THE SOLES

Application: Deficiency of vital energy and essence.

Steps: Sit with the feet stretched. Pull the toes of the left foot with the left hand, and rub the left sole with the right hand till it feels warm. Take 24 deep breaths, and direct *qi* throughout the body. Repeat on the other side. (Figure 15.17)

GE XIANWENG RELIEVING THE CHEST

Application: Depression in the chest.

Steps: Stand splayfooted, and interlace the fingers. Rub the chest left and right with the palms a number of times. Take 24 deep breaths, and direct *qi* throughout the body. (Figure 15.18)

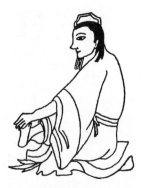

Figure 15.17
Xue Daoguang Rubbing the Soles

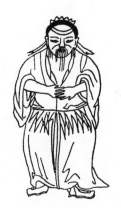

Figure 15.18
Ge Xianweng Relieving the Chest

Wang Yuyang Dispelling Pain

Application: Pain all over due to cold.

Steps: Stand upright, with the left foot in front of the right. Clench both fists, and hold them on the abdomen. Take 24 deep breaths, and direct *qi* throughout the body. Reverse the position of the feet and repeat the whole process. (Figure 15.19)

Ma Gu Removing Stasis

Application: Obstructed circulation of *qi*.

Steps: Stand. If the circulation of *qi* is obstructed in the left part of the body, raise the right forearm to the horizontal level. Clench the right fist, and point to the right with the index finger. Take five deep breaths, and direct *qi* through the left part of the body. If the obstruction occurs on the right side, repeat the movement and breathing on the opposite side. (Figure 15.20)

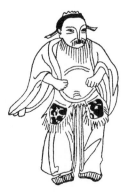 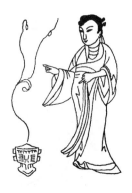

Figure 15.19
Wang Yuyang Dispelling Pain

Figure 15.20
Ma Gu Removing Stasis

Zhang Guolao Adding and Subtracting Heat

Application: Dim vision due to upward invasion of excessive blood heat at the *sanjiao* (triple burner, three visceral cavities housing the internal organs).

Steps: Sit up, cross-legged. Rub the *dantian* till it is warm. Then press the palms on the knees, and sit still with the mouth closed till the breath calms down. Take nine deep breaths, and direct *qi* throughout the body. (Figure 15.21)

Chen Zide's Sleeping Exercise

Application: Typhoid fever.

Steps: Lie on one side, and curl up the legs. Rub the hands together till they are hot, and hold the genitals. Take 24 deep breaths, and direct *qi* throughout the body. (Figure 15.22)

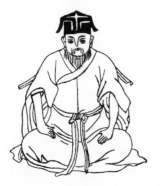

Figure 15.21
Zhang Guolao Adding and
Subtracting Heat

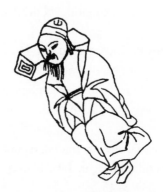

Figure 15.22
Chen Zide's Sleeping Exercise

SHI XINGLIN WARMING THE DANTIAN

Application: Coldness and pain in the abdomen due to hernia.

Steps: Sit up, and rub the hands together till they are hot. Cover the *dantian* with the hands. Take 49 deep breaths, and direct *qi* throughout the body. (Figure 15.23)

HAN XIANGZI REVIVING THE HEART

Application: Bent waist and uncontrollable shaking of the head.

Steps: Stand, and bow low until the fingertips touch the toes. Take 24 deep breaths, and direct *qi* throughout the body. (Figure 15.24)

GODDESS ZHAOLING DRIVING AWAY DISEASE

Application: Cold, numbness and pain in the legs and feet.

Steps: Standing, point the left index finger straight to the front. Pinch the inside of the left forearm with the right hand. Take 24 deep breaths, and direct *qi* throughout the body. (Figure 15.25)

LÜ CHUNYANG PREVENTING ALL DISEASES

Application: All diseases.

Method One: Seated erect, press the acupoints behind the ears, nine times on each side. Take nine deep breaths, and direct *qi* throughout the body.

Method Two: Press the hands upon the knees, and turn the upper body left and then right. Take 14 deep breaths, and direct *qi* throughout the body. (Figure 15.26)

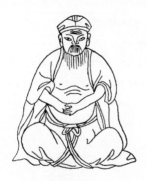

Figure 15.23
Shi Xinglin Warming the *Dantian*

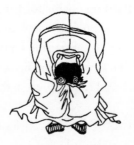

Figure 15.24
Han Xiangzi Reviving the Heart

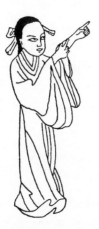

Figure 15.25
Goddess Zhaoling Driving Away Disease

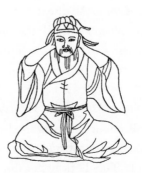

Figure 15.26
Lü Chunyang Preventing All Diseases

CHEN XIYI IMITATING A RECLINING OX WATCHING THE MOON

Application: Spermatorrhea, awake or asleep.

Steps: Lie on one side with the legs curled up. When the semen is about to slip out, put the left index finger into the right nostril, and press the end of coccyx with the right middle finger to contain the semen. Take six deep breaths, and direct *qi* throughout the body. (Figure 15.27)

LORD FUYOU DRAWING A SWORD

Application: All heart pains.

Steps: Adopt a T-stance with the feet. Stretch the left hand towards the left lower front, and pose the right hand as if about to draw a sword. Meanwhile, turn the head to the left, and fix the eyes in the same direction. Take nine deep breaths, and direct *qi* throughout the body. Then change sides and repeat. (Figure 15.28)

XU SHENZU SHAKING HIS NECK

Application: All diseases of the head, face, shoulders and back.

Steps: Sit straight with the palms up and fingers overlapped in front of the chest just below the heart. Shake the neck left and right. Take 24 deep breaths on each side alternately. (Figure 15.29)

CHEN NIWAN DISPELLING HEADACHE

Application: Dizziness and headache.

Steps: Sit straight, and embrace the ears and the back of the neck with the hands. Take 12 deep breaths, and direct *qi* throughout the body. Put the palms together 12 times. (Figure 15.30)

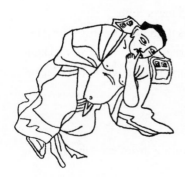

Figure 15.27
Chen Xiyi Imitating a Reclining Ox
Watching the Moon

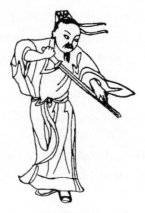

Figure 15.28
Lord Fuyou Drawing a Sword

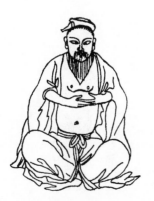

Figure 15.29
Xu Shenzu Shaking His Neck

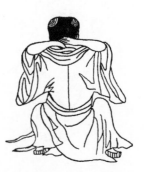

Figure 15.30
Chen Niwan Dispelling Headache

Cao Guojiu Kicking off His Boots

Application: Pains in the abdomen and lower limbs.

Steps: Stand, and pose the right hand as if pressing against a wall. Let the left arm hang down naturally. Kick the right foot forward as if kicking off a boot. Take 16 deep breaths, and direct *qi* throughout the body. Repeat on the reverse side. (Figure 15.31)

Cao Xiangu Gazing at the Taiji Diagram

Application: Sore and swollen eyes resulting from excessive internal heat.

Steps: Press the tongue tip against the maxilla, and gaze at the tip of the nose. Imagine directing the internal heat down to the insteps, and the essence in the kidneys to the top of the head. Take 36 deep breaths as if leading the excessive heat out of the mouth. Repeat the whole process three times. (Figure 15.32)

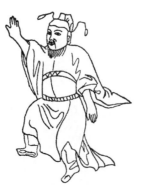

Figure 15.31
Cao Guojiu Kicking off His Boots

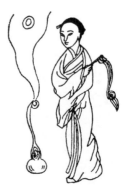

Figure 15.32
Cao Xiangu Gazing at the Taiji Diagram

Yin Qinghe Sleeping Method

Application: Weak spleen and stomach, and indigestion.

Steps: Lie on the back with the left knee bent. Prop up the straight right leg with the left knee. Pull the shoulders toward the belly with the hands. Take six deep breaths, and direct *qi* throughout the body during the pulling process. (Figure 15.33)

Sun Xuanxu Mimicking a Dragon Stretching its Claws

Application: Pains in the waist and legs.

Steps: Sit and stretch out the legs straight forward. Pull the tiptoes toward the body with the hands. Take 19 deep breaths, and direct *qi* throughout the body during the pulling process. (Figure 15.34)

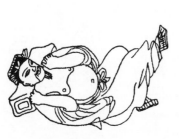

Figure 15.33
Yin Qinghe Sleeping Method

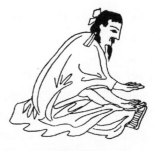

Figure 15.34
Sun Xuanxu Mimicking a Dragon
Stretching its Claws

Gao Xiangxian Imitating a Phoenix Spreading its Wings

Application: Pains in the waist and legs.

Steps: Stand, and bow. Let the clenched fists hang down naturally. Rise on the toes, and open the fists. Raise the hands above the head by way of the sides of the head, and breathe out gently three to four times through the mouth and nose. Pose the right foot behind the left one, right toes against the left heel. Lower the arms, with the left hand pointing towards the rear upper left and the right hand towards the front lower right, like a phoenix spreading its wings. Look in the direction of the right hand. Take 10 deep breaths, and direct *qi* throughout the body. (Figure 15.35)

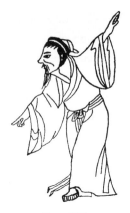

Figure 15.35
Gao Xiangxian Imitating a
Phoenix Spreading its Wings

Fu Yuanxu Hugging His Head

Application: Dizziness.

Steps: Sit straight, and rub the hands together till they are warm. Place one hand over the other just on the very top point of the head. Close the eyes, and concentrate the mind. Breathe through the mouth so that the warm air rises to the top of the head. Then take 17 deep breaths, and direct *qi* throughout the body. (Figure 15.36)

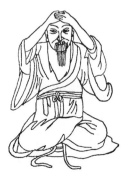

Figure 15.36
Fu Yuanxu Hugging His Head

130

Li Hongji Playing with the Moon

Application: Disharmony between *qi* and blood, and abnormal ascent of *qi*.

Steps: Cross the limbs, left over right, and press the hands and feet on the ground. Take 12 deep breaths, and direct *qi* throughout the body. Then cross the limbs in the opposite direction, and repeat the process. (See Figure 15.37)

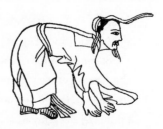

Figure 15.37
Li Hongji Playing with the Moon

Li Tieguai Leaning on His Crutch

Application: Pains in the waist and back.

Steps: Hold a crutch with both hands, and prop the left side of the waist on it. Lean on the crutch, and take 108 deep breaths in three groups of 36 breaths each, and direct *qi* throughout the body. Kneel, but ensure that the knees do not touch the ground. Sway the body to the left and right several times. Then prop the right side of the waist on the crutch, and repeat the whole process. (Figure 15.38)

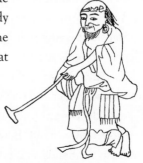

Figure 15.38
Li Tieguai Leaning on His Crutch

Immortal Yuzhen Soothing His Kidneys

Application: Leg pain.

Steps: Sit upright, and clench both fists. Rub the fists together till they are warm. Then rub Jingmen, the two soft areas in the lower back, taking 24 deep breaths. (Figure 15.39)

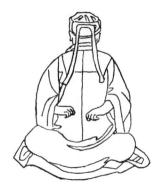

Figure 15.39
Immortal Yuzhen Soothing
His Kidneys

Li Yepu Paying Homage to Guanyin

Application: Leg pain.

Steps: Sit upright, and straighten the legs. Press the roots of the thighs with the hands, and direct vital *qi* to the lower limbs. Meditate while taking 12 deep breaths. (Figure 15.40)

Lan Caihe Imitating a Dragon Swinging its Horns

Application: Pains throughout the body.

Steps: Sit upright, and straighten the legs. Clench both fists, and extend them forward horizontally. Press the thumb sides of the fists against each other and bow the head. Move the upper body forward, and take 24 deep breaths.

Alternative: Stand. Bow the head. Pull the toes with the hands, and take 24 deep breaths. (Figure 15.41)

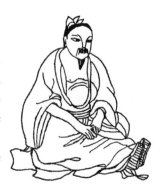

Figure 15.40
Li Yepu Paying Homage
to Guanyin

Liu Xigu Imitating a Tiger Exhibiting its Power

Application: Dysentery with purulent and bloody stools.

Steps: Stretch the right arm forwards and the left arm backwards. Clench the right fist, with the index and middle fingers extended forwards. Stretch the left hand backwards, fingers extended and parted, and palm down. Place the right foot in front and the left foot behind, turning the face to the left and looking in that direction. Reverse the positions of the feet and hands. Proceed on both sides alternately. Take nine deep breaths on the left for dysentery with purulent stools and nine breaths on the right for dysentery with bloody stools. (Figure 15.42)

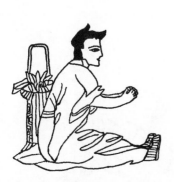

Figure 15.41
Lan Caihe Imitating a Dragon
Swinging its Horns

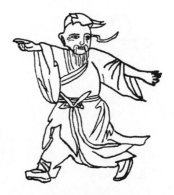

Figure 15.42
Liu Xigu Imitating a Tiger
Exhibiting its Power

ZHANG WUMENG STANDING ON ONE FOOT

Application: Pain throughout the body.

Steps: Stand straight, and raise the left arm. Clench the left fist, with the index and middle fingers extended and pointing upward. Half-clench the right fist, and point it downwards. Suspend the left foot in the air while turning the face to the right and looking in that direction. Take nine deep breaths. Change to the other side, and repeat. (Figure 15.43)

XIA YUNFENG IMITATING A CROUCHING DRAGON

Application: Pains in the back.

Steps: Crouch on the ground, supported on the hands and knees. Turn the head to the right, and take six deep breaths. Then do the same on the left. (Figure 15.44)

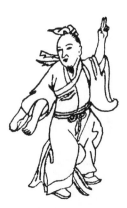

Figure 15.43
Zhang Wumeng Standing on
One Foot

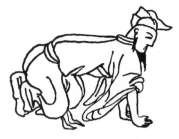

Figure 15.44
Xia Yunfeng Imitating a Crouching Dragon

Hao Taigu Holding Up the Sky

Application: Bloated stomach and abdomen.

Steps: Sit upright, cross-legged, and raise both hands as if holding the sky up. Take a deep breath, and direct *qi* upwards. Repeat nine times. Then take another deep breath, and direct *qi* downward. Again, repeat nine times. (Figure 15.45)

Sun Bu'er Waving a Flag

Application: Bloated stomach and abdomen.

Steps: Stand straight. Bow the upper body forward, both hands extended forward as if reaching for something. Bend the right knee, and raise the right foot backward repeatedly, taking 24 breaths. Do the same with the left foot. (Figure 15.46)

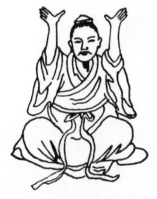

Figure 15.45
Hao Taigu Holding Up the Sky

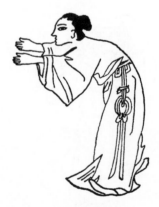

Figure 15.46
Sun Bu'er Waving a Flag

Chang Tianyang Paying Homage to Guanyin

Application: Heart pains in the chest and back.

Steps: Stand splayfooted, and touch the chin to the chest. Interlace the fingers, and press the hands on the abdomen. Take 19 deep breaths. (Figure 15.47)

Dongfang Shuo Massaging His Big Toes

Application: Hernia.

Steps: Sit upright, with both feet stretched out. Massage the big toes with both hands. Take five deep breaths, and direct vital *qi* in the abdomen throughout the body.

Alternative: Massage all the toes repeatedly to produce a better effect. (Figure 15.48)

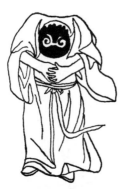

Figure 15.47
Chang Tianyang Paying
Homage to Guanyin

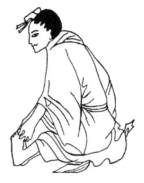

Figure 15.48
Dongfang Shuo Massaging
His Big Toes

Peng Zu Improving His Eyesight

Application: Dim eyesight.

Steps: Sit with both palms propped on the ground and the fingertips pointing behind. Stretch out the right leg while bending the left one. Place the right leg upon the left foot. Take five deep breaths to circulate *qi* in the lungs to remove rheumatic pains and colds. Persistent practice may allow you to see in the dark as clearly as in the daylight.

Alternative: In the hours between one and three in the morning, when the rooster crows, sit upright. Rub the palms together, and then apply them to the eyes. Repeat three times. This method improves the eyesight, leading to shining eyes. (Figure 15.49)

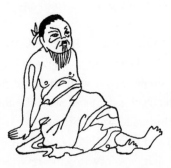

Figure 15.49
Peng Zu Improving His Eyesight

137

XVI

DAOYIN EXERCISES OF ANCIENT IMMORTALS

The illustrations in this section are based upon those in the second volume of the three-volume *Chi Feng Sui*, or *Marrow of the Crimson Phoenix*, compiled by Zhou Lüjing of the Ming Dynasty in 1579. Altogether, 46 pictures were reprinted in this book, based on the 16th-century block-printed edition of *Chi Feng Sui*. Most names mentioned in the captions are those of immortals in ancient Chinese mythology.

WO QUAN FLYING AFTER A GALLOPING HORSE

Application: Dysentery with purulent and bloody stools.

Steps: Stand with the right foot in front and the left one behind. Clench the right fist, with the index and middle fingers extended and pointing forward. Stretch the left hand horizontally backwards, palm up and fingers slightly curved as if holding something. Take a step with the left foot forward, and reverse the position and gesture of the hands. Proceed on both sides alternately. Take nine breaths on each side as you do so. (Figure 16.1)

HUANG SHIGONG PRESENTED WITH A SHOE

Application: Leg pains.

Steps: Sit with both legs stretched out. Press the roots of the thighs with the hands. Meditate while taking 12 deep breaths. (Figure 16.2)

JIAN KENG LOOKING INTO A WELL

Application: Waist and leg pains.

Steps: Stand firm, with both fists clenched. Lean forward until the fists touch the ground. Then rise up slowly, raising the hands above the head. Take 12 gentle breaths through the nose, with the mouth shut. (Figure 16.3)

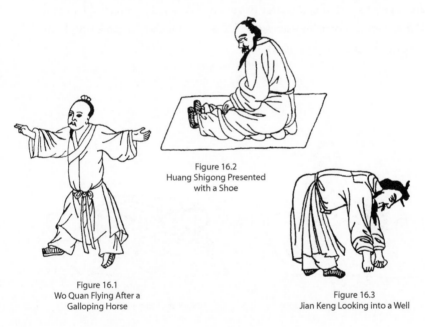

Figure 16.2
Huang Shigong Presented
with a Shoe

Figure 16.1
Wo Quan Flying After a
Galloping Horse

Figure 16.3
Jian Keng Looking into a Well

Xiao Fu Mending Shoes in a Market

Application: Spermatorrhea and premature ejaculation.

Steps: Sit with both legs stretched out. Clasp the sole of the right foot with both hands as tightly as possible. Take three deep breaths on the left and four on the right. (Figure 16.4)

Qiong Shu Using a Rock for a Pillow

Application: Spermatorrhea.

Steps: Lie on the right side, with the legs curled. Block the left nostril with the fingers of the right hand, and press the end of the coccyx with the left fingers to curb the discharge of semen. Take six deep breaths. Control your semen reservoir by exercising the above steps when semen is about to be discharged. (Figure 16.5)

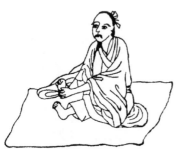

Figure 16.4
Xiao Fu Mending Shoes in a Market

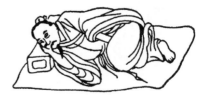

Figure 16.5
Qiong Shu Using a Rock for a Pillow

JIE YU SINGING MADLY

Application: Waist pains.

Steps: Stand firm. Prop the right hand and right foot against a wall, leaving the left hand hanging naturally. Take 18 deep breaths. Repeat on the left side. (Figure 16.6)

JUAN ZI FISHING AT HEZE

Application: Chronic furuncles (boils or carbuncles).

Steps: Sit upright, cross-legged. Prop the left fist against the left flank, and place the right palm upon the right knee. Concentrate the mind in meditation. Take six deep breaths, and direct *qi* to the furuncles. Reverse the position and gesture of the hands, and repeat. (Figure 16.7)

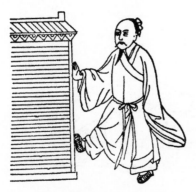
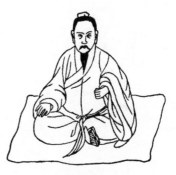

Figure 16.6
Jie Yu Singing Madly

Figure 16.7
Juan Zi Fishing at Heze

Rong Chenggong Guarding the Valley Spirit in Tranquillity

Application: Dizziness.

Steps: Sit upright. Clench the teeth gently, and hold the breath for a moment. Cover the ears with the palms. Cross the index finger over the middle finger of each hand and flip hard on the occiput with the index finger slipping off the middle finger as if striking a drum. Repeat 36 times on each side. Then click the teeth 36 times. (Figure 16.8)

Zhuang Zhou's Butterfly Dream

Application: Nocturnal emission.

Steps: Lie on the right side with the head resting on the right palm. Straighten the left leg, and bend the right one. Meditate and take 24 deep breaths. (Figure 16.9)

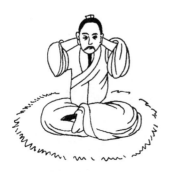

Figure 16.8
Rong Chenggong Guarding
the Valley Spirit in Tranquillity

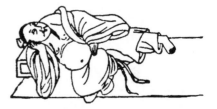

Figure 16.9
Zhuang Zhou's Butterfly Dream

DONGFANG SHUO ABANDONING HIS DIRECTOR'S CAP

Application: Cold and giddiness.

Steps: Sit upright. Press Fengchi (the two depressions behind the neck) with the middle three fingers of both hands. Cover the ears with the palms and interlace the fingers at the back of the head. Take 12 deep breaths, and direct *qi* throughout the body. (Figure 16.10)

KOU XIAN PLAYING THE ZITHER

Application: Rheumatic headache and obstructed circulation of blood and *qi*.

Steps: Sit cross-legged with the palms on the knees. Turn the neck and shoulders to the left, and take 12 deep breaths. Repeat on the right side. This exercise is called "shaking the heavenly pillar." (Figure 16.11)

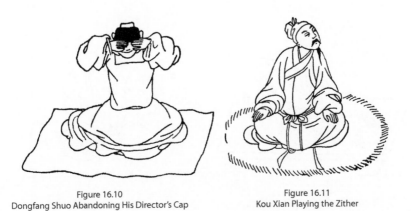

Figure 16.10
Dongfang Shuo Abandoning His Director's Cap

Figure 16.11
Kou Xian Playing the Zither

Xiu Yanggong Lying on a Stone Bed

Application: Typhoid.

Steps: Lie on the left side, knees bent. Rub the palms together. Then cover the right ear with the right palm, and hold the penis with the left hand. Take 24 deep breaths. (Figure 16.12)

Wang Zijin Playing the *Sheng*

Application: All diseases.

Steps: Sit upright, cross-legged. Massage the Zhongfu point (about 3 cm below the outer end of the shoulder blade, in the first intercostal space, on either side). Repeat nine times taking nine deep breaths. This will clear the Ren Meridian, and remove all diseases. (Figure 16.13)

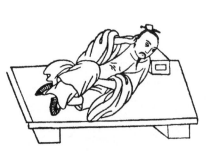

Figure 16.12
Xiu Yanggong Lying on a Stone Bed

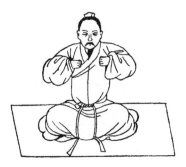

Figure 16.13
Wang Zijin Playing the *Sheng*

ZHONGLI YUNFANG MASSAGING HIS KIDNEYS

Application: Weakness and cold in the kidneys area and pain in the waist and legs.

Steps: Sit upright, cross-legged. Rub the hands until they are warm, and clench the fists. Massage Jingmen, the two softest areas in the lower back, with the backs of the hands. Take 24 deep breaths. (Figure 16.14)

LORD DONGHUA LEANING ON A STICK

Application: Pain in the waist and back.

Steps: Stand straight, leaning on a stick held in one hand. Turn the neck and waist left and right, and take 18 breaths on either side, one breath every three turns. Then kneel down, still leaning on the stick. Turn the neck and waist left and right several times before the knees reach the ground. (Figure 16.15)

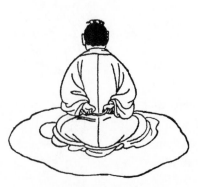

Figure 16.14
Zhongli Yunfang Massaging His Kidneys

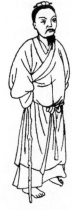

Figure 16.15
Lord Donghua Leaning on a Stick

Shan Tu Pulling His Feet

Application: Nocturnal emission.

Steps: Sit with both legs stretched out. Clasp the soles of the feet with both hands, and take nine deep breaths. (Figure 16.16)

Xu Jingyang Slaying Demons with a Flying Sword

Application: Stomachache.

Steps: Stand with the feet forming a T-shape. Raise the right hand, and turn the upper body to the left. Place the left hand on the small of the back, and take nine deep breaths. Change to the other side, and repeat. (Figure 16.17)

Wei Boyang Preaching Taoism

Application: Pain in the shoulder, back and arms.

Steps: Sit upright with the right leg extended and the left leg bent. Raise the left arm to shoulder height, with the left palm erect and facing the left. Massage the abdomen with the right hand, and take 12 deep breaths. Change to the other side, and repeat. (Figure 16.18)

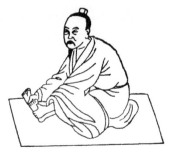

Figure 16.16
Shan Tu Pulling His Feet

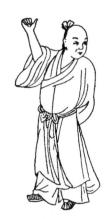

Figure 16.17
Xu Jingyang Slaying Demons
with a Flying Sword

Zi Zhu Loosening His Hair and Playing the Zither

Application: Obstructed circulation of blood and *qi*, imbalanced *yin* and *yang* in the internal organs, dim sight, dizziness and weakness.

Steps: Sit upright and cross-legged, and rub the soles of the feet until they feel warm. Then place the palms on the knees. Take nine deep breaths through the mouth. (Figure 16.19)

Dragon Swishing its Tail

Application: Waist pain.

Steps: Stand, bow and touch the toes. Take 24 deep breaths. (Figure 16.20)

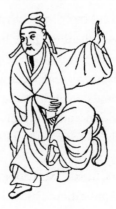

Figure 16.18
Wei Boyang Preaching Taoism

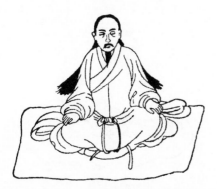

Figure 16.19
Zi Zhu Loosening His Hair and Playing the Zither

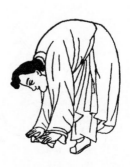

Figure 16.20
Dragon Swishing its Tail

Fu Lü Meditating with Eyes Closed

Application: Pain in the abdomen, and inability to conserve energy.

Steps: Sit upright, cross-legged. Embrace the lower abdomen with the hands, and close the eyes. Concentrate the mind in meditation. Take 49 deep breaths. (Figure 16.21)

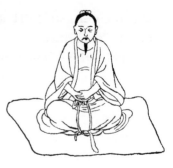

Figure 16.21
Fu Lü Meditating with
Eyes Closed

Tao Chenggong Riding a Dragon

Application: Distension and depression in the chest.

Steps: Sit upright, cross-legged. Raise the arms on the left side while turning the head to the right. Take nine deep breaths. Repeat on the opposite side. (Figure 16.22)

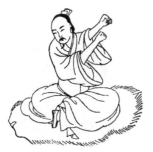

Figure 16.22
Tao Chenggong Riding a Dragon

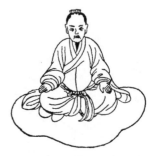

Figure 16.23
Gu Chun Sitting on the City Gate

Gu Chun Sitting on the City Gate

Application: Diseases of the internal organs.

Steps: Sit upright, cross-legged. Press the hands upon the knees, and turn the upper body left and right. Take 14 deep breaths. (Figure 16.23)

Xie Ziran Sitting Cross-legged on the Sea

Application: Fatigue.

Steps: Sit upright, cross-legged. Prop the fists hard against the flanks in line with the pit of the stomach. Meditate while taking 24 deep breaths. (Figure 16.24)

Song Xuanbai Lying in the Snow

Application: Indigestion.

Steps: Lie flat on the back, and massage the chest and stomach repeatedly. Take six deep breaths. (Figure 16.25)

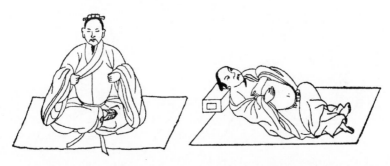

Figure 16.24
Xie Ziran Sitting Cross-legged on the Sea

Figure 16.25
Song Xuanbai Lying in the Snow

MA ZIRAN FALLING DRUNK INTO THE ZHA RIVER

Application: Dry cholera.

Steps: Lie on the abdomen, with the legs raised. Stretch the arms backwards and upwards. Take 12 deep breaths. (Figure 16.26)

XUAN SU HAVING NO SHADOW

Application: Spermatorrhea.

Steps: Sit upright. Massage the sole of the left foot with the thumbs while taking 24 deep breaths. Change to the sole of the right foot, and repeat. (Figure 16.27)

FU JU POLISHING BRONZE MIRRORS

Application: Pain throughout the body.

Steps: Sit upright, fists and legs stretched forward. Extend the upper body forward along with the fists. Take 12 deep breaths. (Figure 16.28)

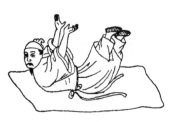

Figure 16.26
Ma Ziran Falling Drunk into
the Zha River

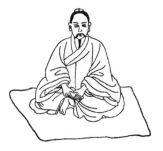

Figure 16.27
Xuan Su Having No Shadow

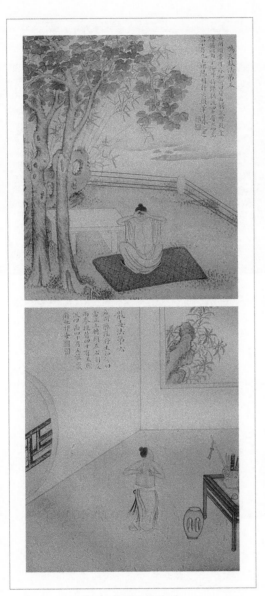

Twelve Massage Methods

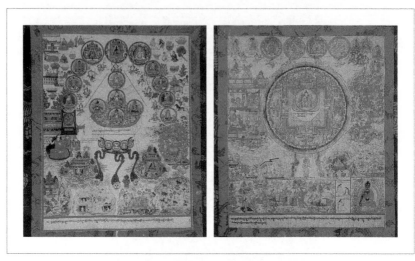

Health Preservation with Tibetan Medicine Illustrated in *The Complete Four-Volume Medical Code Wall Chart Series*

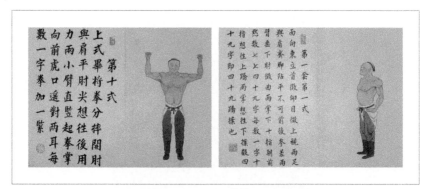

Qi-Regulating Exercises to Foster Exterior Vigor

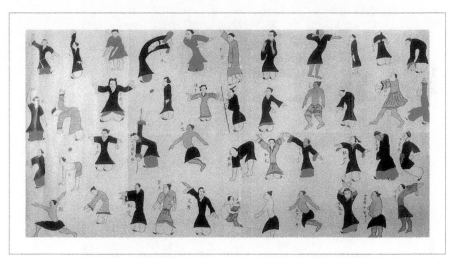

Picture of *Daoyin* Physical and Breathing Exercises

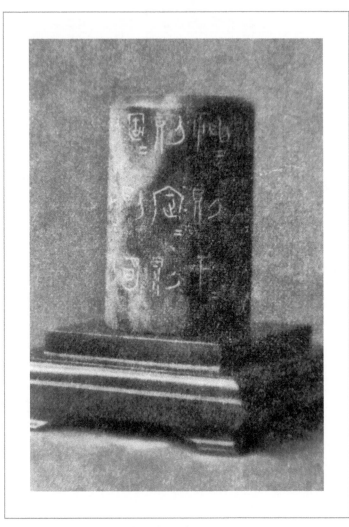

Jade Pendant with Inscription
Describing *Qi* Circulation

Lü Chunyang Directing *Qi*

Application: Pain in the back and arms.

Steps: Stand and stretch the left arm forward. Pinch the muscular parts of the left forearm with the right hand, taking 22 deep breaths. Repeat on the right arm. (Figure 16.29)

Han Zi Searching for a Dog in the Mountains

Application: Paralysis.

Steps: Stand, with the fingers of the left hand pointing left. Turn the head right, and take 24 deep breaths. Repeat on the other side. (Figure 16.30)

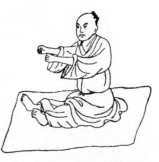

Figure 16.28
Fu Ju Polishing Bronze Mirrors

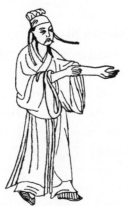

Figure 16.29
Lü Chunyang Directing *Qi*

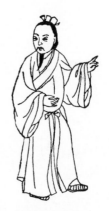

Figure 16.30
Han Zi Searching for a Dog in
the Mountains

151

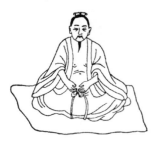

Figure 16.31
Qiu Xuanjing Ascending to
Heaven on Clouds

QIU XUANJING ASCENDING TO
HEAVEN ON CLOUDS

Application: Weakness, cold and pain in the small intestine.

Steps: Sit upright, cross-legged. Rub the *dantian* with both hands while taking 49 deep breaths. (Figure 16.31)

HE XIANGU PINNING A FLOWER
IN HER HAIR

Application: Dizziness.

Steps: Sit upright, and embrace the back of the head with the interlaced fingers. Take 17 deep breaths. (Figure 16.32)

HAN XIANGZI RESERVING QI

Application: Decline of blood and *qi*.

Steps: Sit cross-legged. Rub the palms together till they are warm, and then wipe the eyes with the palms. Prop the fists against the flanks, and direct the vital *qi* upwards. Take 24 deep breaths. (Figure 16.33)

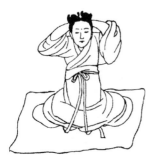

Figure 16.32
He Xiangu Pinning a Flower
in Her Hair

CAO GUOJIU PLAYING THE CLAPPERS

Application: Paralysis.

Steps: Sit upright with the right leg stretched forward and the left leg bent. Cup one hand in the other in front of the chest, and move the arms left while looking to the right. Take 24 deep breaths. Repeat on the other side. (Figure 16.34)

HOU DAOXUAN MAKING A BOW

Application: Pains in the chest and back.

Steps: Stand splayfooted, and place the chin on the chest. Raise the hands along the abdomen, and fold them before the chest. Take 17 deep breaths. (Figure 16.35)

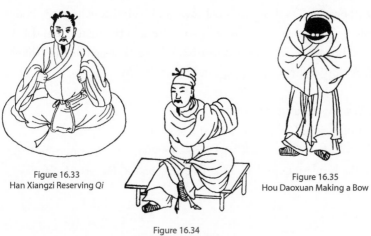

Figure 16.33
Han Xiangzi Reserving *Qi*

Figure 16.34
Cao Guojiu Playing the
Clappers

Figure 16.35
Hou Daoxuan Making a Bow

Xuan Zhenzi Sitting on Water and Reciting Poems

Application: Distended stomach and abdomen.

Steps: Sit upright, cross-legged. Raise both hands as if holding something, and take nine deep breaths. Lower the hands, and take another nine deep breaths. (Figure 16.36)

Xu Que Pinning Flowers in His Hair

Application: Distended abdomen and pain throughout the body.

Steps: Stand firm with the fists half-clenched. Raise the fists above the head, and shift the center of gravity to the heels. Contract the anus, and take nine deep breaths. (Figure 16.37)

Liu Hai Playing with the Golden Toad

Application: Typhoid with tightness and pain throughout the body.

Steps: Stand firm, with the left foot in front of the right one and arms akimbo but some distance from the body. Take 12 deep breaths. Change the position of the feet, and repeat. (Figure 16.38)

Bai Yuchan Circulating Qi

Application: Distended chest and stomach.

Steps: Sit cross-legged. Clasp each shoulder with the opposite hand. Turn the head and eyes left. Take 12 deep breaths. (Figure 16.39)

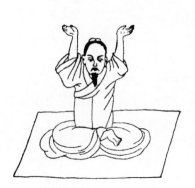

Figure 16.36
Xuan Zhenzi Sitting on Water and
Reciting Poems

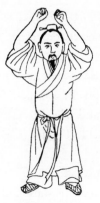

Figure 16.37
Xu Que Pinning Flowers
in His Hair

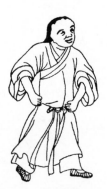

Figure 16.38
Liu Hai Playing with the
Golden Toad

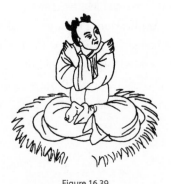

Figure 16.39
Bai Yuchan Circulating *Qi*

Lan Caihe Singing in the Street

Application: Obstructed circulation of blood and *qi*.

Steps: Stand. Raise the left hand forward if obstruction occurs on the left side. Circulate *qi* on the left side, and take 18 deep breaths. Repeat on the right side. (Figure 16.40)

Lingyang Ziming Angling

Application: Pain in the waist and legs.

Steps: Sit with the arms and legs stretched forward. Move the upper body back and forth slowly while taking 19 deep breaths. (Figure 16.41)

Wu Tongwei Meditating

Application: Prolonged hookworm disease.

Steps: Sit upright with the hands on the knees. Meditate while holding the breath. Move *qi* all over the body 19 times so that blood and *qi* circulate smoothly. (Figure 16.42)

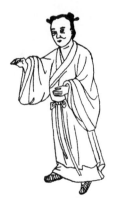

Figure 16.40
Lan Caihe Singing in the Street

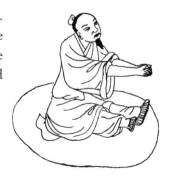

Figure 16.41
Lingyang Ziming Angling

Zi Ying Grabbing a Fish

Application: Disordered circulation of blood and *qi*.

Steps: In a standing position, bow and grasp the toes of each foot with the opposite hand. Sway the body left and right. Circulate *qi* 12 times on each side. (Figure 16.43)

Chen Xiyi Sleeping Soundly on Mount Huashan

Application: Depletion of blood and *qi* due to excessive sexual activity.

Steps: Lie on the right side with the head resting on the right hand. Clench the left fist, and massage the abdomen back and forth with it. Bend the right leg slightly, and place the left foot in front of the right thigh. Regulate the breath, and meditate. Circulate *qi* while taking 12 deep breaths. Long practice of this exercise enriches blood and *qi*. (Figure 16.44)

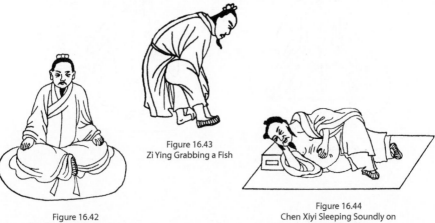

Figure 16.43
Zi Ying Grabbing a Fish

Figure 16.42
Wu Tongwei Meditating

Figure 16.44
Chen Xiyi Sleeping Soundly on
Mount Huashan

Jin Keji Sitting Enveloped by Incense

Application: Unbearable cramp caused by dry cholera.

Steps: Sit upright. Clasp the knees with the hands, and stamp on the ground with alternate feet, nine times each side. Circulate *qi* 24 times. (Figure 16.45)

Qi Xiaoyao Sitting Alone

Steps: Sit upright. Massage the small of the back and flanks with the backs of the hands. Circulate *qi* 32 times. (Figure 16.46)

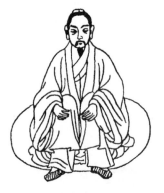

Figure 16.45
Jin Keji Sitting Enveloped in Incense

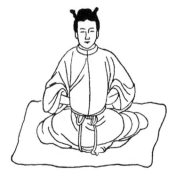

Figure 16.46
Qi Xiaoyao Sitting Alone

XVII

NINE-STEP EXERCISE FOR PROLONGING LIFE

Nine-step Exercise for Prolonging Life was compiled by Fang Kai, who lived in the reigns of Emperor Kangxi (r. 1662–1722) and Emperor Qianlong (r. 1723–1735) of the Qing Dynasty. Fang Kai was accomplished in *daoyin* exercises for preserving health, and compiled the *Illustrated Exercises for Massaging the Abdomen and Circulating Qi*. The manuscript was later illustrated, captioned and published by Bai Yanwei, who renamed it *Prolonging Life in Nine Steps*. The book consists of nine drawings, each illustrating a step of *daoyin* exercise. It is stated in the book that *yin* and *yang* are the vital forces for the production and transformation of the body, and the imbalance of *yin* and *yang* should be rectified through *daoyin* exercises. The method of massaging the abdomen removes stagnancy through movement and advances movement in stillness. Consistent with the principles of *yin* and *yang* and the theory of the Five Elements, it can stimulate the life force, eliminate diseases and prolong life.

The Nine-step Exercise for Prolonging Life is also clearly explained and vividly illustrated in Volume 16 of *An Illustrated Book of Exercises to Benefit the Internal Organs—Promoting the Metabolism, Limbering Up the Tendons and Refreshing the Marrow* by Zhou Shuguan of the late Qing Dynasty. That book instructs that massage of the abdomen should proceed from the rim to the center of the abdomen, and stipulates the best time for doing the exercise, number of times and other points for attention. The instructions are as follows: Massaging the abdomen requires concentration and peace of mind. One should lie straight on one's back on a flat bed with a low pillow, legs side by side, and massage the abdomen gently and slowly. Completion of each of the first eight steps once in sequence is counted as one session. Each course consists of seven consecutive sessions and the finishing movement of sitting up and turning the upper body 21 times. The exercise should be practiced regularly three times a day, namely, after waking up in the morning, at noon and before sleeping in the late evening. Both the morning and evening sessions are imperative, but the noon session may be omitted if inconvenient. The exercise progresses step by step, twice each session at the beginning, five three days later and seven after another three days. It is suitable for all except pregnant women. The illustrations in this book are based on those in the 1930 litho-printed edition of *An Illustrated Book of Exercises to Benefit the Internal Organs—Promoting the Metabolism, Limbering Up the Tendons and Refreshing the Marrow.*

Step 1: Massage the pit of the stomach from the left clockwise in 21 circles with the middle three fingers of both hands. (Figure 17.1)

Step 2: Massage from the pit of the stomach downwards to the pelvis with the middle three fingers of both hands. (Figure 17.2)

Step 3: Massage from the pelvis towards the sides, and then upwards by the sides of the navel with the middle three fingers of both hands until the hands meet at the pit of the stomach. (Figure 17.3)

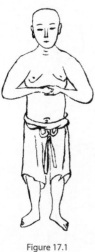 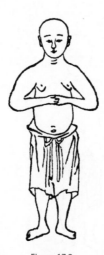 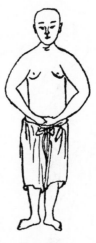

Figure 17.1
Step 1

Figure 17.2
Step 2

Figure 17.3
Step 3

Step 4: Massage between the pit of the stomach and the pelvis back and forth 21 times with the middle three fingers of both hands. (Figure 17.4)

Step 5: Massage around the navel from the left clockwise in 21 circles with the right hand. (Figure 17.5)

Step 6: Massage around the navel from the right clockwise in 21 circles with the left hand. (Figure 17.6)

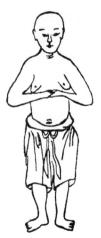

Figure 17.4
Step 4

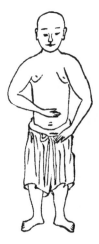

Figure 17.5
Step 5

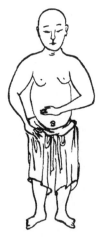

Figure 17.6
Step 6

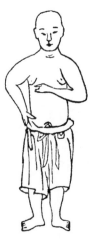

Figure 17.7
Step 7

Step 7: Hold the left side of the waist with the left hand, thumb front and fingers behind. Massage from below the left breast downwards to the root of the left thigh 21 times with the middle three fingers of the right hand. (Figure 17.7)

Step 8: Hold the right side of the waist with the right hand, thumb front and fingers behind. Massage from below the right breast downwards to the root of the right thigh 21 times with the middle three fingers of the left hand. (Figure 17.8)

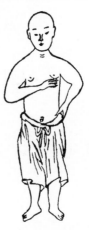

Figure 17.8
Step 8

Step 9: After the massaging, sit up, cross-legged. Place the hands on the knees, and press the thumbs against the inside of the knees. Bend the toes slightly. Turn the upper body 21 times from the left, to the front, to the right, and backwards, and then another 21 times in the reverse direction. When turning left, extend the breast and shoulders further left than the left knee; when turning forwards, bend the upper body to the knees; when turning right, extend the breast and shoulders further right than the right knee; when turning backwards, lean back, and bend the back. Turn slowly and easily. (Figure 17.9)

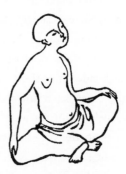

Figure 17.9
Step 9

XVIII

FACE MASSAGE EXERCISE

The illustrated text of Face Massage Exercise is incorporated in Volume 1 of *The Essence of Longevity* compiled by Xu Wenbi in 1771 (see Chapter IV). The exercise enhances the facial appearance through self-massage. The illustration is based on one in the 1775 block-printed edition of *The Essence of Longevity*.

Immediately after waking up in the morning (or at any other time), open the eyes slowly. Rub the backs of thumbs together till they feel hot, and then massage the eyelids with them, nine times on each side. Close the eyes, and move the eyeballs left and right alternately, nine times on each side. Shut the eyes tightly for a while, and then open them. Move the eyeballs left and right alternately, nine times on each side. This step dispels rheumatic fever and eliminates eye diseases forever.

Rub the backs of the thumbs together till they feel hot, and then massage the nose with the two thumbs moving in opposite directions, altogether 36 times. This step nourishes the lungs.

Press the outer corners of the eyes with the end joints of the thumbs, 36 times on each side. Then repeat on the inner corners of the eyes. This step enhances the eyesight.

Rub the palms together till they feel hot, and then massage the face from top to bottom 90 times. Make sure to cover every part of the face. Wet the palms with saliva, and rub them together till they feel warm. Then massage the face 90 times, as above. This step lightens the face and prevents the emergence of freckles and wrinkles.

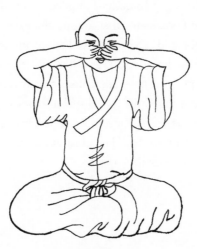

Figure 18.1
Face Massage Exercise

XIX

INTERNAL EXERCISE

The Internal Exercise is recorded in Volume 2, Internal Exercises for Cultivation, of *The Essence of Longevity* compiled by Xu Wenbi in 1771 (see Chapter IV). The book states that among the exercises which are wholesome and harmless and can be practiced by anyone, at any time and anywhere, the Breath-Regulating and Yellow River Reverse-Flow Exercises are simple and easy to practice, have miraculous curative effects, and only require a calm mind and calm breath to dispel diseases and prolong life. This chapter introduces the Yellow River Reverse-Flow Exercise, also known as the Small Circulation of the Tao. The illustrations are based on those in *The Essence of Longevity* compiled by Xu.

FIGURE 19.1

At midnight or 2 pm every day, first calm the mind, and then take off the clothes and sit upright, cross-legged, with fists clenched and eyes and mouth shut (Figure 19.1). Concentrate the mind, and concentratedly examine the internal organs. Click the teeth 36 times. Prop the tip of tongue against the upper tooth ridge behind the teeth till saliva accumulates. Rinse the mouth with the saliva, and swallow it loudly. Examine the internal organs, and send the saliva forcefully down to the *dantian*.

FIGURE 19.2

As Figure 19.2 shows, imagine heat in the *dantian*, and gently send the heat to the tip of the coccyx, and then up through the kidneys, Jiaji, Shuangguan, Tianzhu and Yuzhen to Niwangong, as if holding back defecation.

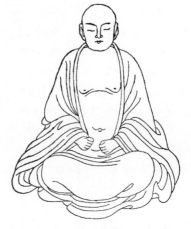

Figure 19.1

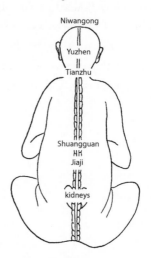

Figure 19.2

167

FIGURE 19.3

Pause for a while, and then prop the tip of the tongue against the upper tooth ridge behind the teeth. Send heat back down from Shenting, through Queqiao, Chonglou, Jianggong, Huangting and Qixue (navel chakra) to the *dantian* (Figure 19.3). Pause for a while, and repeat the three steps three times.

Then regulate the breath, click the teeth and swallow saliva. Sit still for a moment. Rub the backs of the thumbs together till they feel hot, and massage the eyes with them. Open the eyes slowly, and massage the body.

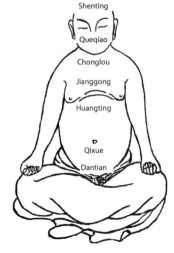

Figure 19.3

XX

EIGHT-SECTION BROCADE EXERCISE FOR PHYSIQUE BUILDING

The Eight-section Brocade Exercise for Physique Building is incorporated in the *Two Classics of Yijin and Xisui* collated by Ma Yizhen in 1843. According to Ma's preface to the book, the two classics of Yijin and Xisui were the doctrines of Bodhidharma, a Mahayana Buddhist who came from India to China in the 6th century and developed the Chinese Chan school of Buddhism. Ma bought many editions of the two classics, and compiled them into one book.

The Eight-section Brocade Exercise for Physique Building refers to the eight steps of physical exercise, namely pulling, grasping, pressing, clenching, pinching, pushing, lifting and drawing. "Practicing the eight steps once each successively in repeated sessions and three times a day persistently ensures a strong physique." The illustrations are based on those in the Youzhu Shanfang edition of the *Two Classics of Yijin and Xisui*.

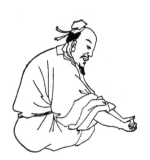

Figure 20.1
First Step—Pulling

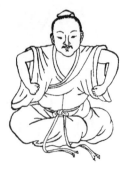

Figure 20.2
Second Step—Grasping

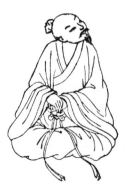

Figure 20.3
Third Step—Pressing

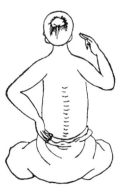

Figure 20.4
Fourth Step—Clenching

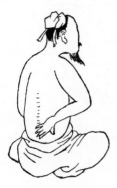

Figure 20.5
Fifth Step—Pinching

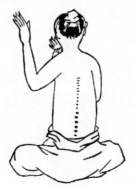

Figure 20.6
Sixth Step—Pushing

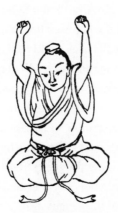

Figure 20.7
Seventh Step—Lifting

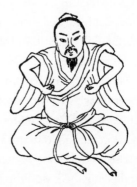

Figure 20.8
Eighth Step—Drawing

XXI

QI-REGULATING EXERCISE TO FOSTER EXTERIOR VIGOR

The *Qi*-Regulating Exercise to Foster Exterior Vigor is recorded in the book *Illustrated Qi-Regulating Exercises to Foster Exterior Vigor* compiled by Tan Fu of the Qing Dynasty and published by Wang Shou.

Little is known about Tan Fu's life. After Wang Shou returned to his hometown in his late years, he restrained himself from carnal desires, and followed a regulated diet to preserve his health and vital *qi* in accordance with Tan Fu's method, and obtained amazing effects. Wang Shou published Tan Fu's book *Illustrated Qi-Regulating Exercises to Foster Exterior Vigor* in 1841.

The book introduces three series of *qi*-regulating exercises, consisting of 22 steps, each step with a colored illustration and a caption (see the color pictures in the center of the book). It starts by bringing forward points for attention, and follows this by describing the stages and functions of the exercise. "The points for attention are as follows: Choose a clean place, and stand facing the East. Prop the tip of the tongue against the upper tooth ridge behind the teeth, and regulate the breath. Raise the face slightly, and look forwards and upwards. Relax the whole body, otherwise *qi* cannot circulate to the fists. Silently count to 49 during each step, and immediately start the next step after each counting period, or *qi* will be interrupted and dissipated. Exert strength only at the hands. The second series must be practiced several days after the first series, and the third, five to seven days after the second. The whole set of exercises can be completed in half a month at the least, and 20 days at most. Sexual intercourse should be avoided in the course of these exercises. Begin to direct *qi* to the vertex after 50 days, and perform a set of exercises seven times within 24 hours, and eat five meals a day for 100 days. A hundred days later, weaker persons will be able to lift 250 kg, and stronger ones 500 kg. The old and weak who are unable to do much labor may practice only the first series, and eat five meals a day to build up their physique and *qi*." The illustrations are based on those of the 1841 block-printed edition of *Illustrated Qi-Regulating Exercises to Foster Exterior Vigor.*

Series I

Step 1: Stand facing the East, head and eyes slightly raised. Position the feet at shoulder width, and align the toes of both feet. Let the shoulders sink, and bend the elbows slightly, palms down and fingers and thumbs pointing forward. Count from one to 49 silently, pushing the fingers and thumbs upwards and pressing the palms down once at the count of each number. (Figure 21.1)

Step 2: Following the previous step, clench the fists, backs of hands forward and thumbs pointing at the thighs. Count to 49 silently, turning the thumbs upwards once at the count of each number. (Figure 21.2)

Step 3: Following the previous step, place the thumbs upon the middle phalanges of the middle fingers. Turn the fists so that the thumbs face forward, and straighten the slightly bent elbows. Count to 49 silently, tightening the fists once at the count of each number. (Figure 21.3)

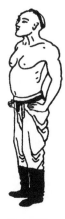
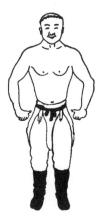
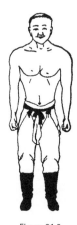

Figure 21.1
Step 1

Figure 21.2
Step 2

Figure 21.3
Step 3

Step 4: Following the previous step, raise the arms vertically to shoulder height, and stretch them forward, with the fists vertical and about 30 cm away from each other, and the elbows slightly bent. Count to 49 silently, tightening the fists once at the count of each number. (Figure 21.4)

Step 5: Following the previous step, raise the arms, fists still clenched, straight into the air, with the thumbs facing each other and slightly apart. Count to 49 silently, tightening the fists once at the count of each number. (Figure 21.5)

Step 6: Following the previous step, lower the fists to about 3 cm from the sides of the ears, elbows in line with the shoulders and the fingers facing forward. Count to 49 silently, tightening the fists once at the count of each number. (Figure 21.6)

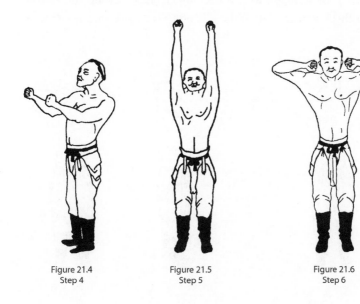

Figure 21.4
Step 4

Figure 21.5
Step 5

Figure 21.6
Step 6

Step 7: Following the previous step, incline the body slightly forward till the heels are just off the ground, and straighten the arms, fists clenched and fingers facing outwards, at shoulder height. Count to 49 silently, tightening the fists once at the count of each number. (Figure 21.7)

Step 8: Following the previous step, move the arms inwards to the same position as in Step 4. Count to 49 silently, tightening the fists once at the count of each number. (Figure 21.8)

Step 9: Following the previous step, draw the fists backward to the height of the collar bones, fingers pointing outwards. Raise the fists to level with the tip of the nose and about 0.5 cm from each other. Count to 49 silently, tightening the fists once at the count of each number. (Figure 21.9)

Step 10: Following the previous step, fling the fists apart, so that the forearms form right angles with the shoulder blades. Strain the elbows back, with the fists aligned with the ears and the fingers forward. Count

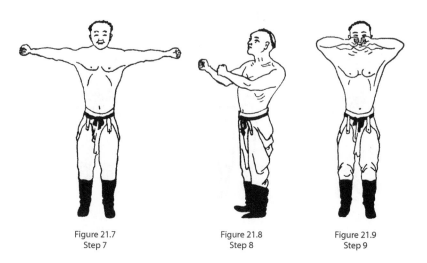

Figure 21.7
Step 7

Figure 21.8
Step 8

Figure 21.9
Step 9

to 49 silently, tightening the fists once at the count of each number. (Figure 21.10)

Step 11: Following the previous step, lower the fists to the level of the navel, with the second knuckles of the index fingers about 0.5 cm away from the navel. Count to 49 silently, tightening the fists once at the count of each number. Take a deep breath, and imagine directing it along with the saliva to the *dantian*. Repeat three times. (Figure 21.11)

Step 12: Following the previous step, unclench the fists, and let the arms hang by the sides. Turn the palms forward, and raise the arms to shoulder height. Lift the heels slightly as an aid to the upward movement. Exert strength as if lifting something heavy, and repeat three times. Then clench both fists, raise them above the head, and fling them downwards. Repeat three times. Kick the left and right feet alternatively, three times on each side. Finally sit still for a while to nourish *qi*. (Figure 21.12)

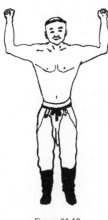 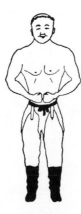 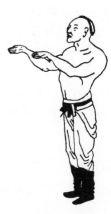

Figure 21.10
Step 10

Figure 21.11
Step 11

Figure 21.12
Step 12

Series II

Step 1: Following Step 11 of Series I, unclench the fists. Turn the palms upward, and raise them to 3 cm above breast height, with the fingertips of one hand 6 to 10 cm away from those of the other. Count to 49 silently. Flatten the palms to the utmost once and imagine directing *qi* to the fingertips at the count of each number. (Figure 21.13)

Step 2: Following the previous step, part the hands horizontally to the sides, and expand the chest. Count to 49 silently, and imagine stretching the hands upwards and backwards at the count of each number. (Figure 21.14)

Step 3: Following the previous step, extend the arms horizontally forwards. Count to 49 silently. Imagine directing *qi* to the fingertips, and protrude the palms slightly upward at the count of each number. (Figure 21.15)

Step 4: Following the previous step, clench the fists, and draw them back to the flanks, with the fingers up and the fists close to the sides. Count to 49 silently, tightening the fists once at the count of each number. (Figure 21.16)

Step 5: Following the previous step, unclench the fists, and push the palms forwards, fingers erect, till the arms are straight. Count to 49 silently, pushing the palms forward and pulling the fingers back at the count of each number. Then repeat Step 11 and 12 of Series I. (Figure 21.17)

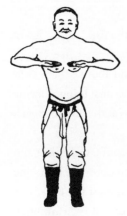

Figure 21.13
Step 1

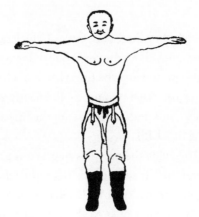

Figure 21.14
Step 2

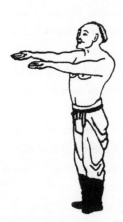

Figure 21.15
Step 3

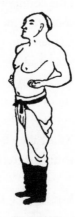

Figure 21.16
Step 4

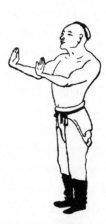

Figure 21.17
Step 5

Series III

Step 1: Following Step 11 of Series I, unclench the fists, palms down, and raise the hands above the chest. Squat down splay-footed, heels about 0.5 cm off the ground and the fingertips of each hand about 0.5 cm away from those of the other. Count to 49 silently while imagining drawing the heels backwards and directing *qi* to the fingertips at the count of each number. (Figure 21.18)

Step 2: Following the previous step, stand up pushing the right palm to the left and the left palm to the right, the left arm upon the right one and the fingers erect. Count to 49 silently, and push the right fingertips to the left and the left ones to the right at the count of each number. (Figure 21.19)

Step 3: Following the previous step, fling the arms apart to shoulder height, palms down. Count to 49 silently. Push out the chest, and stretch the hands upwards and back at the count of each number. (Figure 21.20)

Step 4: Following the previous step, move the arms with the elbows bent to the front of the chest, the left hand above the right, and the left palm facing left and the right palm facing right. Count to 49 silently, while imagining directing *qi* to the fingertips at the count of each number, without the arms touching the body. (Figure 21.21)

Step 5: Following the previous step, let the arms hang down at the sides, and turn the palms to face the back, elbows and fingers slightly bent. Count to 49 silently while imagining directing *qi* to the fingertips at the count of each number.

Then repeat Step 11 and 12 of Series I. Finally, sit still facing East for a while. (Figure 21.22)

Direction of *qi* to the vertex can only start after 50 days of practice. In the squatting posture in Step 1 of Series III, stare upwards, clench the teeth, turn the head left and right three times, and imagine directing *qi* to the vertex. Directing *qi* to the lower body after 60 days of practice can strengthen the lower parts of the body.

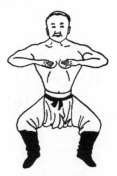

Figure 21.18
Step 1

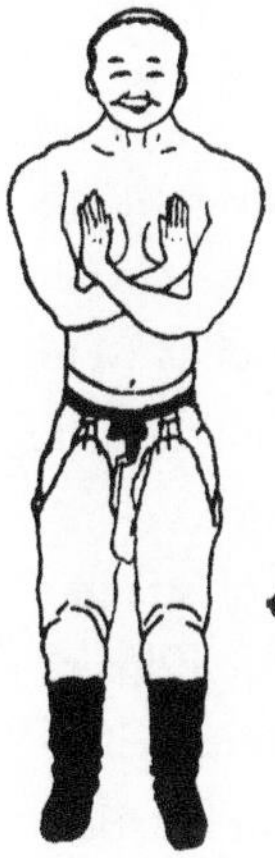

Figure 21.19
Step 2

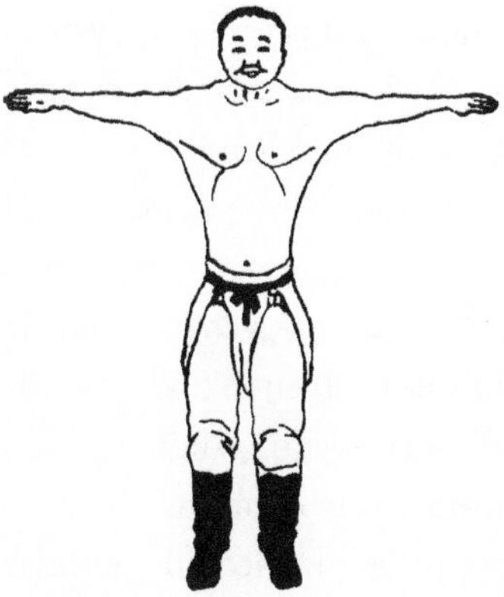

Figure 21.20
Step 3

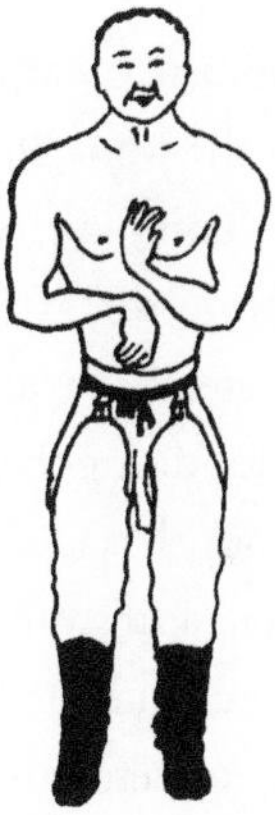

Figure 21.21
Step 4

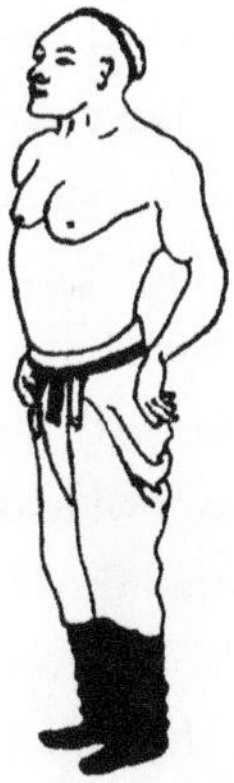

Figure 21.22
Step 5

XXII

BREATH-GULPING EXERCISES FOR REMOVING DISEASES

The illustrations for the breath-gulping exercises for removing diseases are based on those in the book *Illustrated Breath-Gulping for Removing Diseases* by an anonymous compiler of the Qing Dynasty. These exercises were transcribed from oral dictation. Furthermore, it adopts the method of gulping breaths instead of training *qi*, and is very easy to practice.

The essentials for doing these exercises are: Stand upright, look straight ahead, open the mouth wide. Then taking a gentle breath, gulp it down, taking vital *qi* with it, as if swallowing water. The gulping sound is inaudible at first, but will grow loud enough to catch the ear with persistent practice. Send *qi* to the *dantian*, returning the vital energy to its source. If the mouth is not wide opened enough, cold wind will enter and harm the body. No extraordinary strength is required, and everything should be done naturally. Alcohol and sex should be avoided at the beginning.

It is advisable for the exercise to be practiced three times every day, namely, in the morning, at noon and in the evening.

The process of coordinated movements and breath-gulping is as follows: Start from the Gentle Forms and gulp seven breaths in all; 10 days later add the Initial Martial Moves, once on each side, gulping six breaths; another 10 days later double the movements; another 10 days later triple the movements, gulping altogether 18 breaths for the Initial Martial Moves; after another 10 days add the Form of Bending over the Knee, and practice it three times on each side, gulping six breaths, and replace the Moon-Watching Forms with the Forms of Fishing for the Moon from the Seabed; 10 days later add the Standing Fighting Forms, once on each side (first left and then right), gulping six breaths. By this time a total of 49 breaths should have been taken in the previous 80 days, so start practicing the Forms of Flapping with a Bag of Grain, and flap all over body (first left and then right); gulp a breath before each flapping—altogether 16 breaths, totaling 65 breaths from the start; one or two months after the start of the Flapping Forms, add the Forms of Crushing Hands and gulp four breaths; 10 days later, add the Forms of Lateral Lift, six breaths, and the Forms of Frontal Lift, three breaths; 10 days later, add the Standing Forms of Xuegong, three breaths; after another 10 days, add the Forms of Lined Elbows, six breaths, a total of 22 breaths since the Flapping Forms. The whole process involves the gulping of 87 breaths.

The *Illustrated Breath-Gulping for Removing Diseases* states at the end that persistent practice of these 60-odd forms alone can dispel diseases and prolong life, and that medicines can only cure diseases in the internal organs, as those in the channels can only be rooted out by practicing the breath-gulping exercises, which soothe the sinews and stimulate blood circulation.

The illustrations are based on the 64 pictures in the 1849 second block-printed edition of the *Illustrated Breath-Gulping for Removing Diseases.*

1. GENTLE FORMS

Horse-Riding Form 1

Stand upright, feet parted at shoulder width and palms facing upwards at the waist without touching the body. (Figure 22.1)

Horse-Riding Form 2

Following the previous form, turn the palms downwards, retaining the position. (Figure 22.2)

Horse-Riding Form 3

Following the previous form, move the hands clockwise horizontally in a circle at the waist. (Figure 22.3)

Horse-Riding Form 4

Following the previous form, push the hands forward, palms and fingers erect and arms at shoulder width and breast height. Gulp a breath, and pause for about the time it takes to gulp three breaths. (Figure 22.4)

Moon-Watching Form 1

Stand upright. Make a leftward lunge, with the left knee bent and right leg straight. Point the left foot forward and to the left, and the right straight forward. The upper body should face forward. Press the left hand upon the left thigh, with the thumb pointing backward. Raise the right hand straight up from the waist to the back of the right ear, and turn it to point downwards, finally forming a hook shape, fingertips pointing backward. (Figure 22.5)

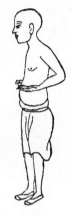

Figure 22.1
Horse-Riding Form 1

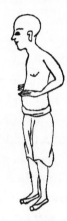

Figure 22.2
Horse-Riding Form 2

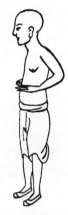

Figure 22.3
Horse-Riding Form 3

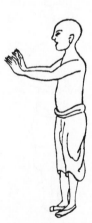

Figure 22.4
Horse-Riding Form 4

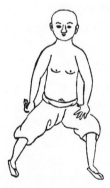

Figure 22.5
Moon-Watching Form 1

Moon-Watching Form 2

Following the previous form, raise the left hand to eye level, and fold the fingers loosely, the thumb in contact with the little finger, the index finger with the ring finger, and the middle finger slightly raised upward. Thus there is formed a hollow between the fingers and the palm. Turn the head to look at a spot between the left hand and elbow. Then turn the head back to the front, and gulp a breath. Turn the head leftwards again to look at a spot between the thumb and the index finger.

Repeat on the other side. Repeat three times on each side, gulping altogether six breaths. (Figure 22.6)

Breath-Smoothing Form 1

The same as Horse-Riding Form 1. (Figure 22.7)

Breath-Smoothing Form 2

Following the previous form, repeat Horse-Riding Form 4 without gulping any breath. (Figure 22.8)

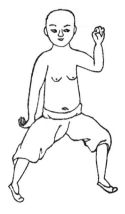

Figure 22.6
Moon-Watching Form 2

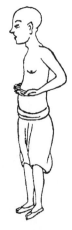

Figure 22.7
Breath-Smoothing Form 1

186

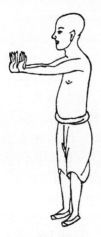

Figure 22.8
Breath-Smoothing Form 2

2. Initial Martial Moves

Initial Martial Moves Form 1

The same as Moon-Watching Form 1. (Figure 22.9)

Initial Martial Moves Form 2 (1)

Following the previous form, raise up the left hand and stretch out horizontally leftward, palm down. (Figure 22.10)

Initial Martial Moves Form 2 (2)

Following the previous form, draw the left hand to the chest. Then stretch it leftward, and draw it back to the chest again. (Figure 22.11)

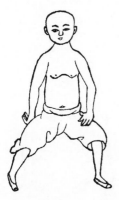

Figure 22.9
Initial Martial Moves Form 1

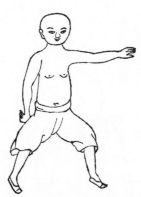

Figure 22.10
Initial Martial Moves Form 2 (1)

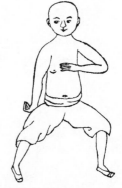

Figure 22.11
Initial Martial Moves Form 2 (2)

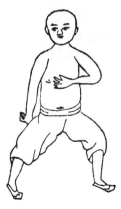

Figure 22.12
Initial Martial Moves
Form 2 (3)

Initial Martial Moves Form 2 (3)

Following the previous form, turn the left palm towards the chest and gulp a breath. (Figure 22.12)

Initial Martial Moves Form 2 (4)

Following the previous form, turn the left palm down, with the hand curved and the middle finger in the highest position. Turn the head to look to the left. (Figure 22.13)

Initial Martial Moves Form 3 (1)

Following the previous form, move the left hand to behind the left ear. Extend the same hand leftwards, palm up, and turn the head to the front. (Figure 22.14)

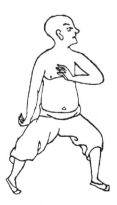
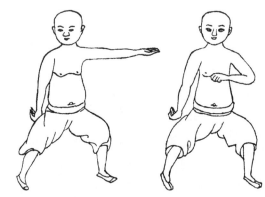

Figure 22.13
Initial Martial Moves
Form 2 (4)

Figure 22.14
Initial Martial Moves
Form 3 (1)

Figure 22.15
Initial Martial Moves
Form 3 (2)

Initial Martial Moves Form 3 (2)

Following the previous form, draw the left hand back to behind the left ear and clench the left fist. Lower this fist to the breast, the back of the hand upward, and gulp a breath. Turn the head to look to the left.

Repeat on the right side. Then repeat three times on each side, gulping altogether 18 breaths. (Figure 22.15)

3. HAND-CRUISING FORM

Stand upright, feet parted at a distance of about 50 cm. Stretch the arms forward, and raise the forearms, fingers parted and palms opposite each other. (Figure 22.16)

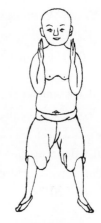

Figure 22.16
Hand-Cruising Form

4. JADE BELT FORM

Following the previous form, cup the backs of the ears with the palms, and then lower them to the sides of the waist at navel height. Point the fingers of one hand at those of the other, with the fingers about 10 cm away from the sides. Gulp a breath. (Figure 22.17)

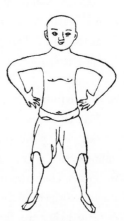

Figure 22.17
Jade Belt Form

5. Waist-Pounding Form

Following the previous form, clench the fists, with the palms up. Gulp a breath. (Figure 22.18)

6. Robe-Lifting Form

Following the previous form, unclench the fists, and turn the hands around at the flanks. Raise the arms slowly forwards and upwards, palms down, as if lifting a weight. Gulp a breath. (Figure 22.19)

7. Head Cover Form

Following the previous form, draw the hands to the flanks, and raise them above the head, palms slanting towards and about 25 cm away from the head. Part the fingers, and let the thumbs hang down at eye height. (Figure 22.20)

8. Face-Rubbing Form

Face-Rubbing Form 1

Following the previous form, hold the palms together, and prop up the chin with the fingertips. Then turn the palms towards the face, the little fingers and forearms side by side, and raise the palms over the forehead. (Figure 22.21)

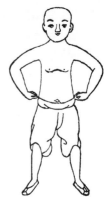

Figure 22.18
Waist-Pounding Form

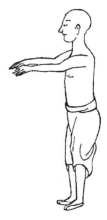

Figure 22.19
Robe-Lifting Form

Face-Rubbing Form 2

Following the previous form, slowly clench the fists, and move them down to beneath the chin. Unclench the fists, and place the thumbs together. Raise the hands over the forehead, and place the little fingers and forearms close together. Again slowly clench the fists, and move them downwards to beneath the chin. (Figure 22.22)

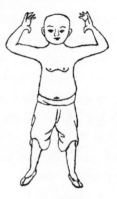

Figure 22.20
Head Cover Form

9. COURT TABLET FORM

Following the previous form, draw the elbows apart, and form a circle with the arms at shoulder height, fists facing each other at a distance of about 60 cm and the backs of the hands up. Gulp a breath. (Figure 22.23)

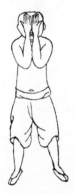

Figure 22.21
Face-Rubbing Form 1

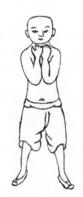

Figure 22.22
Face-Rubbing Form 2

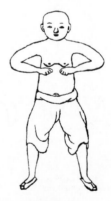

Figure 22.23
Court Tablet Form

10. Lateral Lifting Forms

Lateral Lifting Form 1

Stand upright, and make a forward left lunge, left knee bent, right leg straight and the upper body leaning over the left knee. Interlace the fingers, and raise the hands over the head. (Figure 22.24)

Lateral Lifting Form 2

Following the previous form, bend the upper body slowly forward, and lower the hands, with the fingers still interlaced, to the left instep. Turn the palms downwards, and then upwards so that the palms meet again. Raise the hands up to between the chin and left knee, and then fling them downwards. Return the upper body to the erect position. (Figure 22.25)

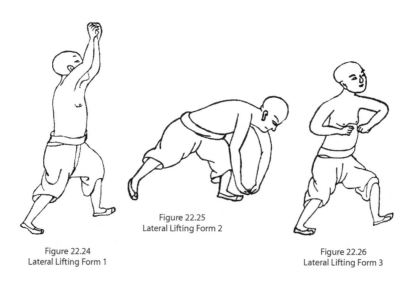

Figure 22.25
Lateral Lifting Form 2

Figure 22.24
Lateral Lifting Form 1

Figure 22.26
Lateral Lifting Form 3

Lateral Lifting Form 3

Following the previous form, unlock the hands, and turn them around the backs of the ears. Form a circle with the arms at shoulder height, fists facing each other at a distance of about 60 cm and the backs of the hands facing up. Gulp a breath. Repeat on the right side. Do three times on each side, altogether gulping six breaths. (Figure 22.26)

11. FRONTAL LIFTING FORMS

Frontal Lifting Form 1

Stand upright, with the feet about 50 cm apart. Interlace the fingers, and raise the hands above the head. (Figure 22.27)

Frontal Lifting Form 2

Following the previous form, bend the upper body slowly forward, and lower the hands to the ground. Turn the palms downwards and then upwards. Raise the interlocked hands to waist height, and fling them downwards. Return the upper body slowly to the erect position. (Figure 22.28)

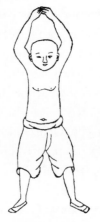

Figure 22.27
Frontal Lifting Form 1

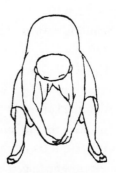

Figure 22.28
Frontal Lifting Form 2

Frontal Lifting Form 3

Following the previous form, unlock the hands, and turn them around the backs of the ears. Clench the fists, and form a circle with the arms at shoulder height, fists facing each other about 60 cm apart and the backs of the hands facing up. Gulp a breath. (Figure 22.29)

Do the Frontal Lifting Forms three times, gulping a total of three breaths.

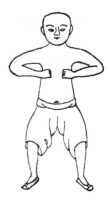

Figure 22.29
Frontal Lifting Form 3

12. Standing Forms of Xuegong

Standing Form 1 of Xuegong

Following the previous form, unclench the fists and straighten the fingers. Raise the hands, and turn them around the backs of the ears. Lower the hands to breast height, palms down. (Figure 22.30)

Standing Form 2 of Xuegong

Following the previous form, lower the hands slowly downward to navel height without any pause during the movement. (Figure 22.31)

Standing Form 3 of Xuegong

Following the previous form, turn the palms upward at the flanks, and raise them up to shoulder height, fingers extended back over the shoulders and thumbs pointing inward in front of the shoulders. (Figure 22.32)

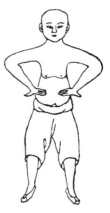

Figure 22.30
Standing Form 1 of Xuegong

Standing Form 4 of Xuegong

Following the previous form, turn the fingers forward, and draw the palms horizontally together at chin height, with the little fingers and wrists side by side. Slowly raise the palms. (Figure 22.33)

Standing Form 5 of Xuegong

Following the previous form, raise the palms above the forehead. (Figure 22.34)

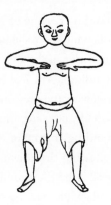

Figure 22.31
Standing Form 2 of Xuegong

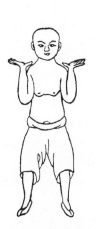

Figure 22.32
Standing Form 3 of Xuegong

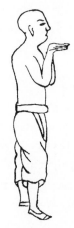

Figure 22.33
Standing Form 4 of Xuegong

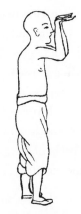

Figure 22.34
Standing Form 5 of Xuegong

Standing Form 6 of Xuegong

Following the previous form, move the palms downward slowly and gradually clench the fists. Lower the fists to chin height. (Figure 22.35)

Standing Form 7 of Xuegong

Following the previous form, open the fists, and straighten the palms horizontally outward, thumbs erect and side by side. (Figure 22.36)

Standing Form 8 of Xuegong

Following the previous form, raise the palms together above the forehead. Part the thumbs, and join the little fingers. Clench the fists gradually while moving them down to chin height. Unclench the fists, and flatten the palms, with the little fingers and wrists side by side. Raise the palms together above the forehead. (Figure 22.37)

Standing Form 9 of Xuegong

Following the previous form, clench the fists gradually while moving them down to chin height. Unclench the fists, and flatten the palms, with the little fingers and wrists side by side. Raise the palms together above the forehead. (Figure 22.38)

Standing Form 10 of Xuegong

Following the previous form, clench the fists gradually while moving them down. Part the fists, and position them in front of the flanks, and then form a circle with the arms, fists facing each other about 60 cm apart and the backs of the hands facing up. Gulp a breath. (Figure 22.39)

Do the Standing Forms of Xuegong three times, gulping three breaths in all.

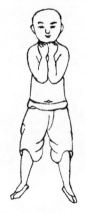
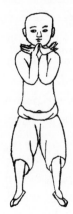
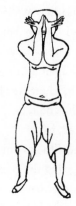

Figure 22.35
Standing Form 6 of Xuegong

Figure 22.36
Standing Form 7 of Xuegong

Figure 22.37
Standing Form 8 of Xuegong

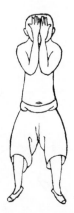
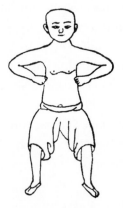

Figure 22.38
Standing Form 9 of Xuegong

Figure 22.39
Standing Form 10 of Xuegong

13. Lined Elbows Forms

Lined Elbows Form 1

Stand upright, and make a leftward lunge, left knee bent and right leg straight. Raise the elbows to chest height. Clench the right fist before the chest, and cup it with the left hand. (Figure 22.40)

Lined Elbows Form 2

Following the previous form, push the left elbow somewhat to the left, and draw it back immediately. Bend the left knee while keeping the right leg straight. Raise the right elbow, with the right fist still in the left hand. (Figure 22.41)

Lined Elbows Form 3

Following the previous form, lift the body as shown in Form 1, with the left knee still bent and right leg still straight. Incline the upper body forward, and gulp a breath. Raise the right elbow, and look at a point about 20 cm in front of the left toes. (Figure 22.42)

Repeat the Lined Elbows Forms on the right side. Repeat three times on each side, altogether gulping six breaths.

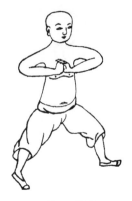

Figure 22.40
Lined Elbows Form 1

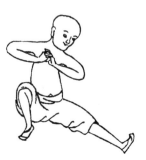

Figure 22.41
Lined Elbows Form 2

198

14. BENDING OVER THE KNEE FORM

Stand upright. Make a leftward lunge, left knee bent and right leg straight. Press the right hand upon the left thigh, about 6 cm above the knee, and put the left hand over the right hand. Incline the upper body forward, with the head facing left. Gulp a breath. Arch the back, and straighten the neck, with the face forward and looking at a point 20 cm ahead of the toes. Do the same on the right side. Repeat three times on each side, gulping six breaths in all. (Figure 22.43)

15. STANDING BATTLE FORMS

Internal Fighting Form 1

Stand upright. Make a leftward lunge, left knee bent, right leg straight, and the upper body facing forward. Raise the left hand to chest height, palm down, and the right hand to navel height, palm up. Oppose the palms, with the fingers straight and parted. Do the same on the right side. (Figure 22.44)

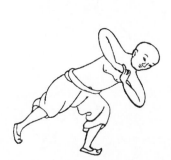
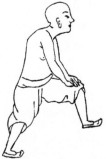
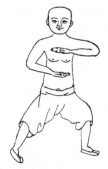

Figure 22.42
Lined Elbows Form 3

Figure 22.43
Bending over the Knee Form

Figure 22.44
Internal Fighting Form 1

Internal Fighting Form 2

Following the previous form, clench the fists, and pull them apart. Draw the left fist to before and about 25 cm from the left breast, thumb inward and fingers downward. Draw the right fist to and about 3 cm from the right flank, thumb outward and fingers upward. Face the front, and gulp a breath. Then turn the head to look to the left. Do the same on the right side. (Figure 22.45)

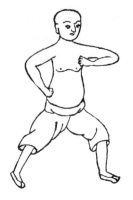

Figure 22.45
Internal Fighting Form 2

Soaring Fist Form

Following the previous form, unclench the left fist. Let the left hand dangle. Then turn the left palm forward, and raise the left hand. Clench the left fist again, and raise it to the front of the forehead, with the fingers facing inward. Face the front, and gulp a breath. Then turn the head to the left, and fix the eyes on the pulse (just below the left wrist). Do the same on the right side. (Figure 22.46)

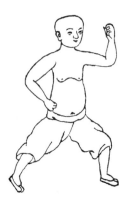

Figure 22.46
Soaring Fist Form

Heart-Piercing Fist Form

Following the previous form, unclench the left fist, and flatten the left palm. Turn the left palm to the right, and move it to behind the left ear. Clench the fist again, and stretch it leftward, with the fingers facing down. Face the front, and gulp a breath. Then turn the head to the left, and fix the eyes on the pulse of the left hand. Do the same on the right side. (Figure 22.47)

Repeat the Standing Battle Forms three times, gulping 18 breaths in all.

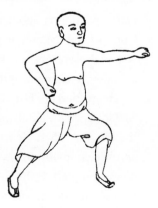

Figure 22.47
Heart-Piercing Fist Form

16. Flapping with a Bag of Grain Forms
Soaring Fist Form 1

Stand upright. Make a leftward lunge, left knee bent and right leg straight. Hold a bag filled with grain in the right hand, and raise the left hand via the left flank. Clench the left fist, and raise the forearm, with the elbow pointing to the left and the upper arm aligned with the shoulder. Gulp a breath. (Figure 22.48)

Soaring Fist Form 2

Following the previous form, hold the bag of grain in the right hand, and with it vigorously flap the inside of the left upper limb to the

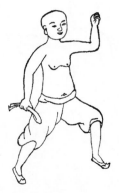

Figure 22.48
Soaring Fist Form 1

palm and fingers about a dozen times or so. Conduct the flapping in sequence, and never reverse. Never go back to make up if some parts are missed. (Figure 22.49)

Heart-Piercing Fist Form

Unclench the left fist, and move it to behind the left ear. Then clench the left fist again, and stretch it leftwards with the fingers facing down. Gulp a breath. Hold a bag of grain in the right hand, and vigorously flap the outside of the left upper limb to the palm and fingers. (Figure 22.50)

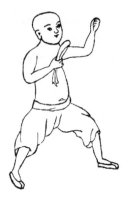

Figure 22.49
Soaring Fist Form 2

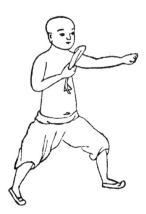

Figure 22.50
Heart-Piercing Fist Form

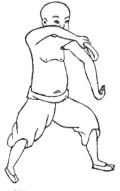

Figure 22.51
Hook Hand Form 1

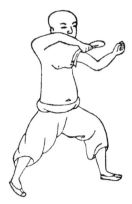

Figure 22.52
Minor Soaring Fist Form

Hook Hand Form 1

Move the left hand to behind the left ear. Then lower it, and pose the hand in a hook shape, fingers pointing backwards. Gulp a breath. Hold a bag of grain in the right hand, and flap the left upper limb from the armpit along the underside of the arm to the little finger. (Figure 22.51)

Minor Soaring Fist Form

Push the left hand forward while clenching the fist. Raise the left fist to a position somewhat lower than in the Soaring Fist Forms. Gulp a breath. Hold a bag of grain in the right hand, and flap from the left shoulder blade via the upper arm to the thumb. (Figure 22.52)

Cauldron-Lifting Form 1

Unclench the left fist and turn it down to the flank. Clench the fist again, and stretch it upward as far as possible, with the fingers facing right. Gulp a breath, fixing the eyes on the left fist. (Figure 22.53)

Cauldron-Lifting Form 2

Following the previous form, hold a bag of grain in the right hand, and flap the left arm from the armpit, along the flank, waist, front side of the thigh, knee, shin and foot, to the toes. (Figure 22.54)

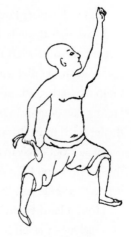

Figure 22.53
Cauldron-Lifting Form 1

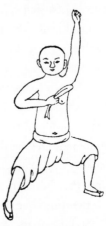

Figure 22.54
Cauldron-Lifting Form 2

Elbow-Turning Form

Unclench the left fist, and put the hand at the back of the left ear. Clench the left fist, and place it parallel with the breast, arm bent. Gulp a breath, and raise the left elbow a little. Hold a bag of grain in the right hand and flap the left arm from the armpit, along the side of the breast, obliquely to the small of the back on the left side, and then via the outside of the left leg, to the ankle and little toe. (Figure 22.55)

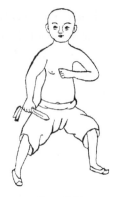

Figure 22.55
Elbow-Turning Form

Hook Hand Form 2

Unclench the left fist and turn it around the back of the left ear. Lower it, and turn the hand into a hook shape, fingers pointing backwards. Gulp a breath. Hold a bag of grain in the right hand, and flap the left side from below the collarbone to the flank. Then flap the abdomen horizontally to the right flank, and transfer the bag to the left hand. Cover the penis with the right hand, and flap the left side of the lower abdomen, and via the inside of the leg to the big toe. Repeat several times to dispel ailments from the abdomen. (Figure 22.56)

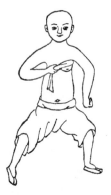

Figure 22.56
Hook Hand Form 2

Bending over the Knee Form 1

Stand upright. Make a leftward lunge, left knee bent and right leg straight. Hold a bag of grain in the right hand, and press it on the middle part of the left thigh. Press the left hand on the bag, and gulp a breath. (Figure 22.57)

Bending over the Knee Form 2

Following the previous form, hold a bag of grain with both hands, and raise it over the top of the head. Bend the arms backwards, and flap the left side of the backbone 20 times. Do not hit the backbone. (Figure 22.58)

Bending over the Knee Form 3

Following the previous form, straighten the left leg, and bend the right knee. Press the right hand on the right thigh, thumb pointing to the left. Incline the upper body backwards and to the right, and fix the gaze on the left knee. Hold a bag of grain in the left hand, and bend the left elbow to flap from the left side of the back to the waist. Turn the left hand around to flap from the left hip, via the back of the left leg, knee and calf to the heel. (Figure 22.59)

Repeat on the right side.

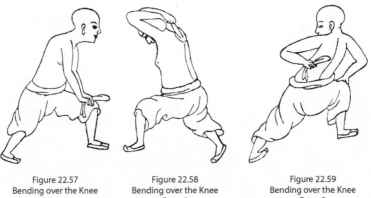

Figure 22.57
Bending over the Knee
Form 1

Figure 22.58
Bending over the Knee
Form 2

Figure 22.59
Bending over the Knee
Form 3

17. Fishing for the Moon from the Seabed Forms

Fishing for the Moon from the Seabed Form 1

Stand upright. Make a leftward lunge, left knee bent and right leg straight. Press the left hand on the left thigh, thumb pointing to the right. Turn the right hand into a hook shape, fingers pointing backwards. (Figure 22.60)

Fishing for the Moon from the Seabed Form 2

Following the previous form, raise the left hand to behind the left ear. Extend the hand to the left, palm forward. (Figure 22.61)

Fishing for the Moon from the Seabed Form 3

Following the previous form, turn the left palm down. (Figure 22.62)

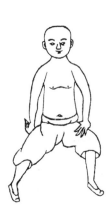

Figure 22.60
Fishing for the Moon from
the Seabed Form 1

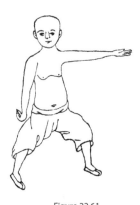

Figure 22.61
Fishing for the Moon from
the Seabed Form 2

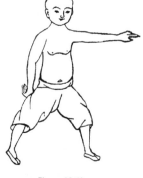

Figure 22.62
Fishing for the Moon from
the Seabed Form 3

Fishing for the Moon from the Seabed Form 4

Following the previous form, bend forward from the waist. Let the left hand hang down, and move it from left to right as if fishing for the moon from the bottom of the sea. Then return to the erect position. (Figure 22.63)

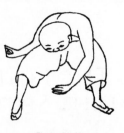

Figure 22.63
Fishing for the Moon from
the Seabed Form 4

Fishing for the Moon from the Seabed Form 5

Following the previous form, raise the left hand to eye level, and fold the fingers loosely, the thumb in contact with the little finger, the index finger with the ring finger, and the middle finger slightly raised upward. Thus a hollow is formed between the fingers and the palm. Gulp a breath. Look at a spot between the thumb and index finger of the left hand. (Figure 22.64)

Repeat the Fishing for the Moon from the Seabed Forms on the right side. Repeat three times on each side, and gulp altogether six breaths.

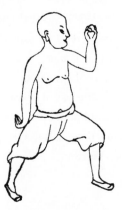

Figure 22.64
Fishing for the Moon from
the Seabed Form 5

XXIII

The 18 Standing Forms in Eight Sections of *Baduanjin*

"The 18 Standing Forms in Eight Sections of *Baduanjin*," seen in the *Illustrations and Techniques of Baduanjin in Standing and Sitting Positions* (*Baduanjin Zuoli Gongtujue*) compiled by Lou Jie of the Qing Dynasty (1644–1911), was first named the "Standing Exercises of *Baduanjin*," and it consisted of 18 forms. In order to distinguish it from the "Standing Forms of *Baduanjin*, it was renamed the "18 Standing Forms in Eight Sections of *Baduanjin*."

Lou Jie was of a weak constitution when he was young, but his health improved after he studied the Standing Exercises of *Baduanjin* under a master named Xu. The following techniques are based on the Fangcao Xuan version.

FORM 1

Keep the body straight, breathe regularly and concentrate the mind. Stand with the feet parallel, and arms relaxed. Thrust out the chest, and suck in the stomach (this applies to every standing form), and slightly bend the arms at the elbows. Keep the hands level, with the palms facing down and the fingertips facing towards the body and about 3 cm away. Part the heels, and then move the toes to the left and right. Then move the heels away from each other again in order to make the toes face slightly inward (keep both feet this way from the beginning to the end of the exercise). Stay immobile for a short while. (Figure 23.1)

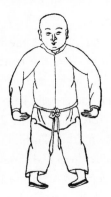

Figure 23.1

FORM 2

After finishing the above form, pause for a second. Then lift the hands up to the rear of the ears, with the palms facing forward. (Figure 23.2)

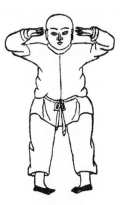

Figure 23.2

FORM 3

After finishing the last form, squat down while pushing the hands forward as hard as you can, with the fingertips brushing the ears. When you crouch, keep the body straight and the crotch level with the knees, in a horse-riding posture. Push both arms straight out at shoulder level and shoulder width. The palms face forward, with the fingers slightly turned up and the distance between the left and right fingertips about 10 cm. (Figure 23.3)

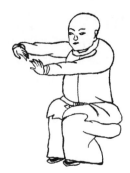

Figure 23.3

FORM 4

As soon as the last form is finished, stretch both hands to the left and right, and then move them downward. The arms remain straight with the fingers curved, as if you are holding a huge rock. (Figure 23.4)

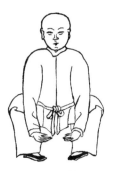

Figure 23.4

FORM 5

As soon as the last form is finished, slowly move the hands up until they reach mouth level, meanwhile raising the body. Keep the shoulders still while moving the hands. (Figure 23.5)

THE FIRST PRINCIPAL FORM—PROPPING UP THE SKY

Turn the palms upward, and separate the hands, with the upper arms level and forearms vertical, and with the palms facing the sky and the fingers facing each other, forming a rectangle. (Figure 23.6)

FORM 6

As soon as the last form is finished, rotate the hands with the palms facing the forehead and the fingers slightly curved, as if holding a heavy object. (Figure 23.7)

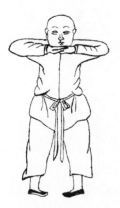 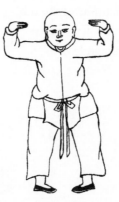 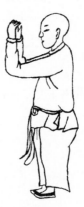

Figure 23.5   Figure 23.6   Figure 23.7

Form 7

Move both hands to cheek level, rotate the hands and push them forward. Crouch as in Form 3. Then repeat forms 4 and 5. When the hands are lifted to mouth level, press the palms downward to make the *qi* descend. That brings the first section to an end. (Figure 23.8)

The Second Principal Form—Drawing a Bow

Move the arms up till they are in line with the shoulders. Turn the head to the left, extend the left hand to the left and crook the right arm as if you are drawing a bowstring. Hold this position for a short while, and then repeat on the right side. In this form, the arms should be level. When the head faces the left, the eyes should focus on the left hand, and when the head faces the right, the eyes should focus on the right hand. (Figure 23.9)

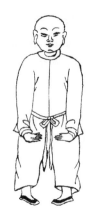

Figure 23.8

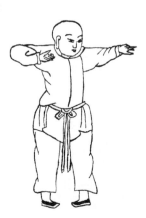

Figure 23.9

FORM 8

As soon as the last form is finished, return the body to an erect position, and extend the arms, with the palms facing forward. Then lift the hands up to the rear of the ears, as in Form 2. Then repeat Forms 3, 4, 5 and 7. This is the end of the second section. (Figure 23.10)

THE THIRD PRINCIPAL FORM—LIFTING A TRIPOD

Repeat Form 5, raising the hands to mouth level. Rotate the left hand up and the right hand down, with the fingers slightly curved. Stretch both arms to the limit. In this form, you should gently stretch the body, and make the eyes look up somewhat. (Figure 23.11)

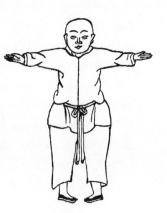

Figure 23.10

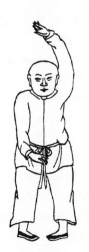

Figure 23.11

213

Form 9

As soon as the last form is finished, rotate both hands quickly, and then slowly move them towards each other, meanwhile squatting down. In this form, when rotating the hands, the eyes focus on the upper hand. Then rise, rotate the right hand up and the left hand down, as in the previous form. (Figure 23.12)

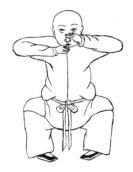

Figure 23.12

At the end of Form 9, move both hands towards each other, rotate the palms, and push outward. Squat as in Form 3, and then repeat Forms 4, 5 and 7.

The Fourth Principal Form—Carrying a Sword

After completing Form 7, move the left arm behind the back, and swing the right arm upward. Turn the head to the left rear, and look at the left heel. Hold this position for a few seconds, then turn the body, swing the left arm upward, place the right hand at the small of the back, turn the head to the right rear, and look at the right heel. This is the form known as "Carrying a Sword." Hold this position for a few seconds, turn the body to the front, stretch the arms, and repeat Forms 2, 3, 4, 5 and 7. (Figure 23.13)

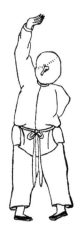

Figure 23.13

The Fifth Principal Form—Squatting like a Gibbon

After Form 7 raise the hands to mouth level. Clench the fists tightly, at the same time crouching, with the fists facing down. Push the fists strongly forward. Rotate and unclench the fists, and draw them back to the chest. Rotate the fists again, and push them forward as before. Repeat this push-and-withdraw movement three times. Unclench the fists, and draw them back to mouth level. Rotate the palms, and push them forward as in Form 3. Repeat Forms 4, 5 and 7. (Figure 23.14)

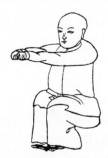

Figure 23.14

Form 10

After Form 7, perform Form 5. Lift up the hands to mouth level, cross the eight fingers (excluding the thumbs), and rotate the palms downward while lifting them up, with the palms still facing down. (Figure 23.15)

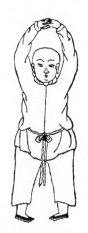

Figure 23.15

215

THE SIXTH PRINCIPAL FORM—CROUCHING LIKE A TIGER

As soon as the last form is finished, bend over, and touch the ground with the fingers interlaced (beginners may simply hold the hands at knee level). This form is known as "crouching like a tiger." After a short while, straighten up slowly, part the hands and raise them to mouth level. Then crouch, and push the palms outward as in Form 3. Repeat Forms 4, 5 and 7. (Figure 23.16)

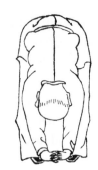

Figure 23.16

THE SEVENTH PRINCIPAL FORM—FLYING SWALLOW

After Form 7, perform Form 5. Then part the hands until the arms are in line with the shoulders, with the palms facing down and the arms slightly leaning backwards. This is the form "flying swallow." After a while, move the hands up to the rear of the ears, as in Form 2. Then repeat Forms 3, 4, 5 and 7. (Figure 24.17)

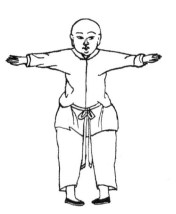

Figure 23.17

The Eighth Principal Form—Standing Horse

With the completion of Form 7, raise the heels and drop them forcefully. Repeat this movement three times. This is the "standing horse" form. After a few seconds, close the eyes and regularize the respiration. Slowly allow the arms to drop. The left foot then kicks towards the right, and the right foot kicks towards the left. Then each foot kicks outward a dozen times. Then swing the hands to the front and back a dozen times. (Figure 23.18)

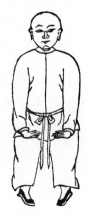

Figure 23.18

XXIV

THE TWELVE SUPPLEMENTARY INTERNAL EXERCISES WITH ILLUSTRATIONS OF *YIJINJING*

The Twelve Supplementary Internal Exercises with Illustrations of *Yijinjing* are taken from the work compiled and edited by Zhou Shuguan of the Qing Dynasty.

In Zhou's preface, he says that he was a sickly child who studied health promotion under a number of teachers. In the fall of 1893 he met Master Jingyi Kongwu in the Temple of Comprehending Wisdom (Tonghui Si) at Ziyang, and was apprenticed to him. The master gave him a book named *An Illustrated Book of Exercises to Benefit the Internal Organs—Promoting the Metabolism, Limbering Up the Tendons and Refreshing the Marrow*, in six volumes. Zhou Shuguan revised it into 17 volumes. Volumes 3 to 14 comprise the main part of the book, generally called the *An Illustrated Book of Exercises to Benefit the Internal Organs—Promoting the Metabolism, Limbering Up the Tendons and Refreshing the Marrow*. Following is a reproduction of 224 illustrations from the 1930 version published by the Chongqing Printing Company.

1. EXERCISES WITH THE BODY FACING THE FRONT

Standing Straight with the Arms Held in an Arc

When practicing this exercise keep the heels close to each other and the balls of the feet rooted to the ground. Turn the left palm upward, and clench the right fist. Put both hands on *huangting* (between the breasts). The knees and spine should be straight. Keep the ears in line with the shoulders and the nose in line with the chest; the eyes should narrow into slits, looking straight at a point about 33 cm in front of you. Clench the teeth, with the tip of the tongue touching the upper palate. Exhale through the nose, and then regulate the breath and calm the *qi* (vital breath); concentrate and take three deep breaths, and then begin to do the next form. (Figure 24.1)

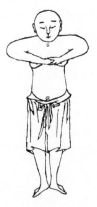

Figure 24.1

Presenting a Pestle

Straighten the back and legs, stretch the spine, with the heels off the ground and the ten toes firmly rooted on the ground. Place the palms together in front of you, with the fingertips in line with the tip of the nose. Take three deep breaths, then push both hands forward, and then do the next form. Refer to the previous form for the requirements for the ears, nose, eyes and teeth. (Figure 24.2)

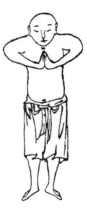

Figure 24.2

Producing the Claws and Displaying the Wings

In this form, push the hands forward as hard as you can, with the palms vertical and the wrists level with the shoulders; keep the palms shoulder width apart. Take three deep breaths, and draw the palms back. Do this form again. (Figure 24.3)

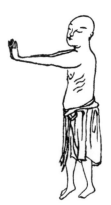

Figure 24.3

Double Phoenixes Salute the Sun

Place the wrists in front of the shoulders, with the tips of the fingers pointing at the sky and the arms at shoulder level. Take three deep breaths, and then part the two palms to the left and right, respectively, of the body. Do this form again. (Figure 24.4)

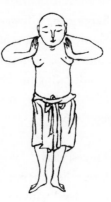

Figure 24.4

The Eagle Spreading its Wings

Push the hands to the sides horizontally, the palms up and the wrists and elbows in line with the shoulders. Breathe deeply three times, and then slowly raise the palms. Do this form again. (Figure 24.5)

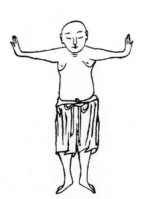

Figure 24.5

Supporting a Tower with Both Hands

Slowly move both hands up over the head, with the palms facing upwards and the back of the hands facing the cavities of the shoulders. Breathe deeply three times. Do this form again. (Figure 24.6)

Three Peaks

Lower the arms by bending the elbows, until they are level with the shoulders and facing outwards. The ten fingers should be separated, with the finger tips pointing to the sky, so as to form "three peaks" (with the head as the central "peak"). Breathe deeply three times. Do this form again. (Figure 24.7)

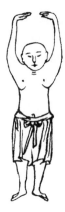

Figure 24.6

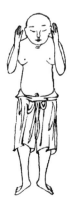

Figure 24.7

The Dragon Sticking Out its Right Claw

Extend the left hand across the chest, and hold the right shoulder blade. Stretch the right hand to the left, as if you are reaching for something. Turn the head, and look in the direction the right hand is pointing in. Then turn the head and eyes to the left to lead the *qi* to the left. Breathe deeply three times. Do this form again. (Figure 24.8)

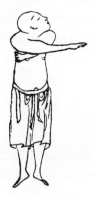

Figure 24.8

The Dragon Sticking Out its Left Claw

The movements of this form are the same as for the previous form, except that they are done in the opposite direction. When sticking out the left hand, turn the head and eyes to the right to lead the *qi* to the right. Breathe deeply three times. Do this form again. (Figure 24.9)

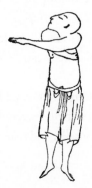

Figure 24.9

Squatting with Arms Held Horizontally

In this form, turn the palms downward, with the fingertips facing each other and in line with the shoulders. Stretch the left arm to the left and the right arm to the right as you breathe deeply once, and squat once. Return to the original form. Repeat this three times. Do this form again. (Figure 24.10)

Circulation of *Qi* Form 1

Interlace the fingers, with the palms facing down. Hold the hands in front of the chest, and take a deep breath. Do this form again. (Figure 24.11)

Circulation of *Qi* Form 2

With the fingers still interlaced, lower the arms until the fingers reach the *dantian*. Take a deep breath. Do this form again. (Figure 24.12)

Circulation of *Qi* Form 3

With the fingers still interlaced, raise the arms in front of the body until they reach shoulder level. Push the palms outward once, with force. Take a deep breath. Do this form again. (Figure 24.13)

Circulation of *Qi* Form 4

Loosen the fingers, stretch the straightened arms to the sides of the body horizontally, and take a deep breath. Do this form again. (Figure 24.14)

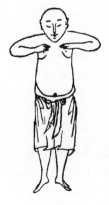

Figure 24.10

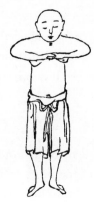

Figure 24.11

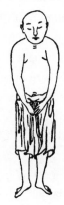

Figure 24.12

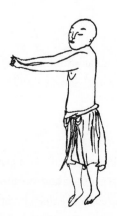

Figure 24.13

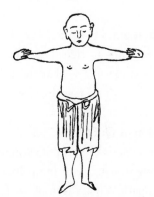

Figure 24.14

Circulation of *Qi* Form 5

Stretch arms out to the sides of the body to the maximum, with both arms kept straight. Cross the ten fingers, with palms facing up; press down the hands hard once and take a deep breath before doing the next form. Do this form again. (Figure 24.15)

Circulation of *Qi* Form 6

Loosen the fingers, and straighten the arms. Raise the arms from the back, passing by the sides of the body, to shoulder level. Interlace the fingers, with the palms facing the chest. Thrust the palms forward forcefully. Take a deep breath. Do this form again. (Figure 24.16)

Circulation of *Qi* Form 7

Rotate the palms outwards, and thrust them forwards forcefully. Do this form again. (Figure 24.17)

Circulation of *Qi* Form 8

Stretch the arms to right and left, respectively, at shoulder height. Bend the wrists inwards so that the palms are facing outwards. Take a deep breath. Do this form again. (Figure 24.18)

Circulation of *Qi* Form 9

Move both hands up from the armpits, past the ears, until both arms are completely straight, with the palms facing each other and no more than 33 cm apart. When the arms are fully extended take a deep breath. Do this form again. (Figure 24.19)

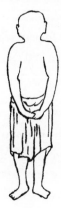

Figure 24.15

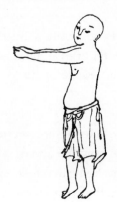

Figure 24.16

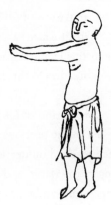

Figure 24.17

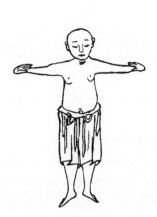

Figure 24.18

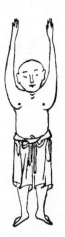

Figure 24.19

Circulation of *Qi* Form 10

With the arms as in the previous position, interlace the fingers, with the palms facing down. Stretch the arms as much as possible, and take a deep breath. Do this form again. (Figure 24.20)

Circulation of *Qi* Form 11

From the previous position, lower the arms in front of the body until they reach shoulder level. The arms are always kept straight, with the fingers interlaced and the palms facing the chest. Extend the arms as far as possible, and take a deep breath. Do this form again. (Figure 24.21)

Circulation of *Qi* Form 12

Rotate the palms outwards. Extend the arms as far as possible, and take a deep breath. Do this form again. (Figure 24.22)

Circulation of *Qi* Form 13

This form is the same as Circulation of *Qi* Form 4. (Figure 24.23)

Circulation of *Qi* Form 14

This form is the same as Circulation of *Qi* Form 5. (Figure 24.24)

Returning to the "Presenting a Pestle" Form

Join the palms in front of the chest, as if praying, with the arms held horizontally at shoulder height. At this point, you have returned to the "Presenting a Pestle" form. Take a deep breath. Do this form again. (Figure 24.25)

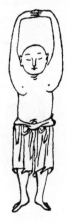

Figure 24.20

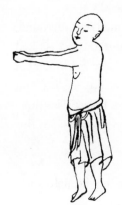

Figure 24.21

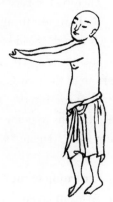

Figure 24.22

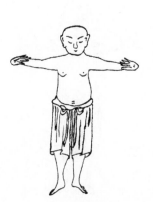

Figure 24.23

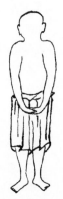

Figure 24.24

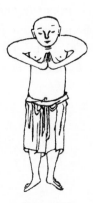

Figure 24.25

229

Turning the Face to the Sky

With the feet firmly planted on the ground, slowly lean the head back until the face is tilted towards the sky. The palms are held together in front of the face. Close the eyes slightly, and visualize the interior of the body. Take three deep breaths to guide the *qi* upwards. Do this form again. (Figure 24.26)

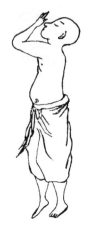

Figure 24.26

Returning to the "Standing Straight with the Arms in an Arc" Form

Return to the "Presenting a Pestle" form. Take a deep breath, hold it, and repeat the "Standing Straight with the Arms in an Arc" form. Take another deep breath, and hold it. Then exhale and inhale to regulate the respiration. (Figure 24.27)

This is the end of the Exercises with the Body Facing the Front.

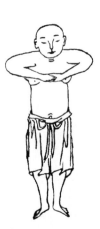

Figure 24.27

2. Exercises with the Body Facing the Side

Supporting the Sky with One Hand

Stand with the feet in a T-shape. Place the left hand on the back of the left hipbone. Raise the right hand from the right hip above the head, with the back of the right hand facing the back of the right foot. At the same time, turn the face towards the sky, with the eyes on the back of the right hand. Concentrate the mind, and take three deep breaths. Guide the *qi* in a reverse direction. Keep the heels, knees and left arm straight without any relaxation. (Figure 24.28)

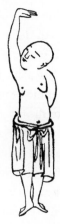

Figure 24.28

Drawing a Sword While Turning the Hand

Move the right hand forcibly around the head clockwise to the left shoulder. Clench the right fist, and take a deep breath to lift the *qi*. Hold the breath. Do this form again. (Figure 24.29)

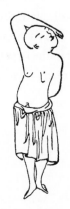

Figure 24.29

Drawing the Bow

Loosen the left hand, and straighten the left arm while raising that arm to shoulder level, with the left palm facing vertically outwards. The feet should be in a T-stance, pointing to the right. Turn the face to the left, root the heels to the ground, and straighten the knees, legs, back and spine. The right arm should be completely bent and at shoulder height. Pull the right hand to the right and push the left hand to the left. The movements of both hands should be coordinated, like drawing a bow. (Figure 24.30)

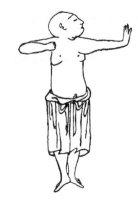

Figure 24.30

Keeping the Shoulders Level

Unclench the fist and stretch both arms horizontally, with the palms facing downward. Raise the heels from the ground. Stretch the arms out to the left and right, respectively. Take a deep breath. (Figure 24.31)

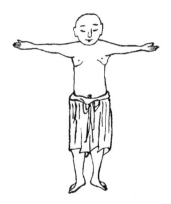

Figure 24.31

White Crane Flaps its Wings

Keeping the heels off the ground and the arms in the previous position, press both palms down while lowering the upper body until it is about 33 cm from the ground. Take a deep breath. Rotate the palms upwards, and lift the arms to shoulder level once more. Repeat this form three times. (Figure 24.32)

Presenting a Pestle and Circulating *Qi*

Stand up after completing the last movements. Join the palms to form the arms in a semi-circle in front of the body (in the "Presenting a Pestle" form), and take a deep breath to circulate *qi*. (Figure 24.33)

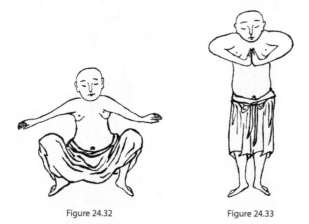

Figure 24.32   Figure 24.33

Turning the Face to the Sky

This form is the same as the "Turning the Face to the Sky" form in the Exercises with the Body Facing the Front on page 230. (Figure 24.34)

Returning to the "Standing Straight with the Arms in an Arc" Form

This form is the same as "Returning to the 'Standing Straight with the Arms in an Arc' Form" in the Exercises with the Body Facing the Front on page 230. (Figure 24.35)

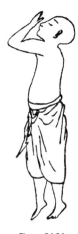

Figure 24.34

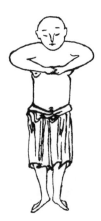

Figure 24.35

3. Squatting Exercises

Presenting a Pestle on a Horse

Squat down as if riding a horse, with the heels off the ground. The rest is the same as the "Presenting a Pestle" form on page 220. (Figure 24.36)

Loosening the Reins

Push the palms forward together, as if giving a horse a loose rein. The lower body assumes the posture of riding a horse. The rest of the form follows the "Presenting a Pestle" form on page 220. (Figure 24.37)

Reining in a Horse

Draw the palms back as if pulling on the reins of a horse. This form resembles that of "Double Phoenixes Salute the Sun." The rest of the form follows that form on page 221. (Figure 24.38)

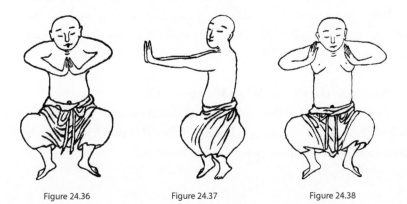

Figure 24.36   Figure 24.37   Figure 24.38

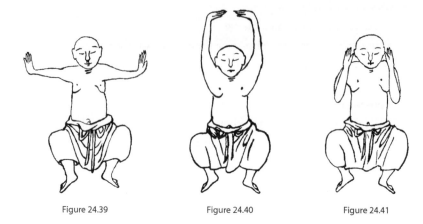

Figure 24.39   Figure 24.40   Figure 24.41

Arranging the Clothes on a Horse

Push the hands to the left and right, respectively, at shoulder height and with the palms vertical and facing outwards. This form resembles that of "The Eagle Spreads its Wings." The rest of the form follows that form on page 221. (Figure 24.39)

Arranging the Helmet While Riding

Rotate the palms to face upwards, and stretch the arms up. This form resembles that of "Supporting a Tower with Both Hands." The rest of the form follows that form on page 222. (Figure 24.40)

Riding with the Wind

Lower the hands with the palms facing outwards just above the shoulder. This form resembles that of the "Three Peaks." The rest of the form follows that form on page 222. (Figure 24.41)

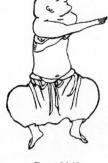

Figure 24.42

Reining to the Left

The movement of the upper body resembles that of the "Dragon Sticks Out its Right Claw" form. The lower body assumes the posture of riding a horse. The respiration, concentration of spirit and the circulation of *qi* are identical to those of the same form. (Figure 24.42)

Reining to the Right

The movement of the upper body resembles that of the "Dragon Sticks out its Left Claw" form. The lower body assumes the posture of riding a horse. The respiration, concentration of spirit and the circulation of *qi* are identical to those of the same form. (Figure 24.43)

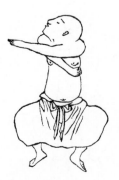

Figure 24.43

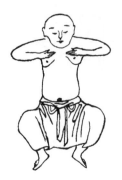

Figure 24.44

Arms Horizontal on Horseback

The movement of the upper body is identical to the form of "Squatting with Arms Held Horizontally." The lower body assumes the posture of riding a horse. The rest of the form follows that form on page 224. (See Fig 24.44)

Resting the Fingers on Top of Each Other on Horseback

With the elbows fully bent and the arms at shoulder level, place the fingers of one hand on the fingers of the other. Take a deep breath. Do the form again. (Figure 24.45)

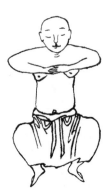

Figure 24.45

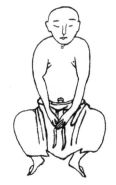

Figure 24.46

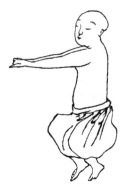

Figure 24.47

238

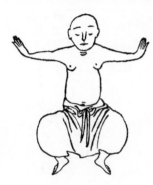

Figure 24.48

Adjusting the Front of the Saddle

Press the hands down to the *dantian* point, with both palms naturally apart and the two arms straight. Take a deep breath. Do the form again. (Figure 24.46)

Casting the Reins to the Front

Stretch the arms to the front at shoulder level and shoulder width apart. Interlace the fingers, and turn the palms to the front, pushing hard at the same time. Take a deep breath. Do the form again. (Figure 24.47)

Separating the Reins to the Left and Right

Push the hands out to the left and right, respectively, with the palms facing outwards. Take a deep breath. Do the form again. (Figure 24.48)

Adjusting the Back of the Saddle

Move the arms to the back of the body. Interlace the fingers, and turn the palms up. Then push the arms down vigorously at the back of the body. Take a deep breath. Do the form again. (Figure 24.49)

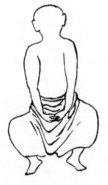

Figure 24.49

Lifting the Reins to the Front

Move the arms to the sides of the body, holding them straight down. Then swing the arms up to the front until they reach shoulder level. Interlace the fingers, with the palms facing the chest, and then push the hands vigorously forward. Take a deep breath. Do the form again. (Figure 24.50)

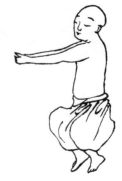

Figure 24.50

Casting the Reins to the Front

Rotate the palms outwards, and push the hands vigorously forwards. Take a deep breath. Do the form again. (Figure 24.51)

Separating the Reins to the Left and Right

Identical to the form with the same name on page 239. (Figure 24.52)

Climbing a Poplar on a Horse Form 1

Move the hands up from the armpits, passing the ears, until the arms are straight, with the palms facing each other and about 33 cm apart. Stretch both hands upwards as hard as you can. Take a deep breath. Do the form again. (Figure 24.53)

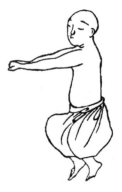

Figure 24.51

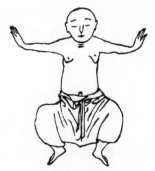

Figure 24.52

Climbing a Poplar on a Horse Form 2

Interlace the fingers, with the palms facing downwards. Stretch the arms firmly upwards. Take a deep breath. Do the form again. (Figure 24.54)

Lifting the Reins to the Front

Lower the arms in the front of the body to shoulder level, keeping them straight. Interlace the fingers with the palms facing the chest. Push the palms vigorously forward. Take a deep breath. Do the form again. (Figure 24.55)

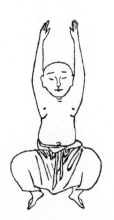

Figure 24.53

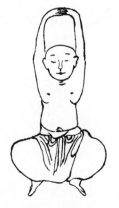

Figure 24.54

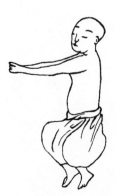

Figure 24.55

Casting the Reins to the Front
Identical to the form with the same name on page 239. (Figure 24.56)

Separating the Reins to the Left and Right
Identical to the form with the same name on page 239. (Figure 24.57)

Adjusting the Back of the Saddle
Identical to the form with the same name on page 239. (Figure 24.58)

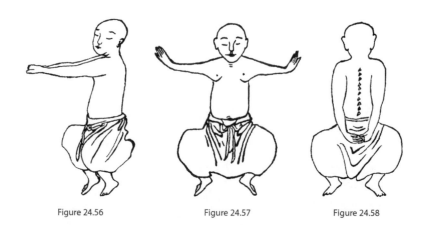

Figure 24.56   Figure 24.57   Figure 24.58

Returning to the "Presenting a Pestle on a Horse" Form

Identical to the "Presenting a Pestle on a Horse" form on page 235. (Figure 24.59)

Standing with the Face Turned to the Sky

Place the heels firmly on the ground, and straighten the legs, knees, back and spine. Take a deep breath. Guide the *qi* up from the toes, past the front of the body, mouth and nose, to the crown of the head; then down along the spine to the sacrum. Then lead the *qi* up in the reverse direction from the sacrum, past the *dantian*, to the head. This is one circle of *qi* movement. Raise the head three times and take three deep breaths, as in the "Turning the Face to the Sky" form on page 230. (Figure 24.60)

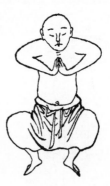

Figure 24.59

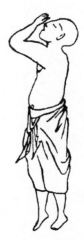

Figure 24.60

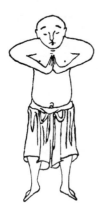

Figure 24.61

Returning to the "Presenting a Pestle" Form

Identical to the form with the same name on page 229. (Figure 24.61)

Returning to the "Standing Straight with the Arms in an Arc" Form

Identical to the form with the same name on page 230. (Figure 24.62)

4. EXERCISES WITH THE BODY INCLINED
Presenting a Pestle on a Horse

Identical to the form with the same name on page 235. (Figure 24.63)

Saluting on a Horse Form 1

In the horse-riding stance, place the palms together, with the fingers touching the bridge of the nose. Take a deep breath. Move the hands up over the crown of the head. Take a deep breath. Stretch the arms firmly over the head. Take a deep breath. Do the form again. (Figure 24.64)

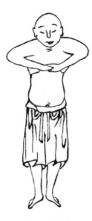

Figure 24.62

Saluting on a Horse Form 2

In the horse-riding stance, lower the hands, with the fingers pointing to the ground, and the arms and back straight and the head upright. Stretch the arms down firmly, with the palms together. Take a deep breath. Then return to the "Presenting a Pestle on a Horse" form and take a deep breath. Continue as for the previous form. (Figure 24.65)

Repeat the above-mentioned first and second forms of "Saluting on a Horse" three times. This means moving the arms up three times and down three times. At this point, the exercise is complete. Every time, the movements and respiration are the same.

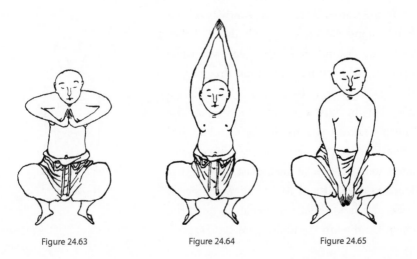

Figure 24.63   Figure 24.64   Figure 24.65

Pushing the Door to the Left and Right

In the horse-riding stance, separate the hands, and move the arms to the sides until they are in line with the shoulders, with the palms facing backwards. Stretch the arms to each side with force, and take a deep breath. Then rotate the palms down, and draw them back horizontally to the sides of the chest. Lift the palms up with force, and take a deep breath. Do the form again. (Figure 24.66)

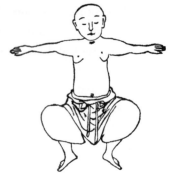

Figure 24.66

Put Three Plates onto the Ground

In the horse-riding stance, slowly lower the hands along the sides of the body until they reach the ground. Keep the head and waist upright, all the fingers touching the ground, the legs bent and the arms straight. Take a deep breath. Raise the hands, and repeat the "Pushing the Door to the Left and Right" form. Practice these two exercises three times alternately. After finishing the last "Pushing the Door to the Left and Right," draw the palms back, and hold them together in front of the chest. Do the form again. (Figure 24.67)

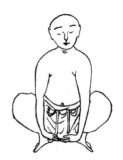

Figure 24.67

Returning to the "Presenting a Pestle" Form
Identical to the form with the same name on page 244. (Figure 24.68)

Turning the Face to the Sky
Identical to the form with the same name on page 230. (Figure 24.69)

Returning to the "Standing Straight with the Arms in an Arc" Form
Identical to the form with the same name on page 230. (Figure 24.70)

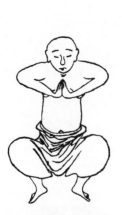

Figure 24.68

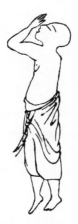

Figure 24.69

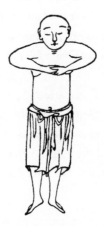

Figure 24.70

5. Exercises with the Body Bent
Presenting a Pestle on a Horse
Identical to the form with the same name on page 235. (Figure 24.71)

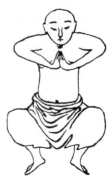

Figure 24.71

Pressing the Ears and Holding the Neck
Hold and press the back of the neck with the three middle fingers of each hand, while at the same time folding the auricles to the front with the bases of the palms. Keep the body straight, and look straight in front of you. Concentrate the mind, and take a deep breath. Do the form again. (Figure 24.72)

Prostration
Slowly press the head down with force to between the knees. Maintain the legs straight and the toes on the ground. Take three deep breaths. Do the form again. (See Figure 24.73)

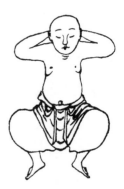

Figure 24.72

Circulating *Qi* in a Reverse Direction

Loosen the palms, and move them from the back of the neck along the sides of the body to the outer sides of the feet, thus bending the body completely. Shift both feet until the toes face each other. The body remains bent, keeping the upper and lower parts of it straight, the head lowered and the spirit concentrated. Take three deep breaths and circulate *qi* in a reverse direction. (Figure 24.74)

Raising the Head and "Wagging the Tail"

Touch the toes with the fingertips, "wag the tail" and raise the head. Concentrate the mind, and fix the eyes. Take three deep breaths. (Figure 24.75)

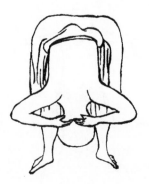 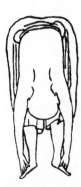 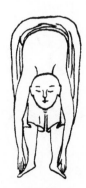

Figure 24.73   Figure 24.74   Figure 24.75

Holding the Palms Together and Calming the Breath

In the horse-riding stance, shift the feet apart, and raise the heels. Lift the body while raising the head; press the palms together, and calm the breath. Take a deep breath. For the rest of this form, see the instructions for the "Presenting a Pestle on a Horse" form on page 235. (Figure 24.76)

Stretching the Arms to Smooth the Veins

In the horse-riding stance, separate the palms to the sides of the body in order to smooth the veins, with the palms facing outwards and the arms in line with the shoulders. Take a deep breath. The other requirements are the same as those for the "Arranging the Clothes on a Horse" form on page 236. (Figure 24.77)

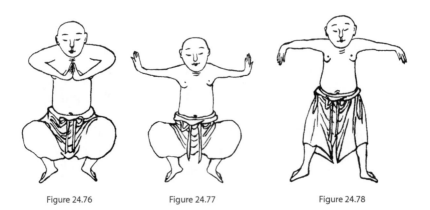

Figure 24.76   Figure 24.77   Figure 24.78

Lifting and Rising

Stand erect, with the legs apart and the arms stretched to either side in line with the shoulders, the hands hanging down and the palms facing inward, as if holding heavy weights. Take a deep breath. (Figure 24.78)

Stamping on Clouds and Dispersing Fog

Stand upright with the legs apart, rotate the palms upwards, and move them up over the head. With both arms straight, cross the palms one in front of the other, and then separate them to the left and right. March on the spot. The rest of the form follows the first form. (Figure 24.79)

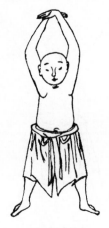

Figure 24.79

Supporting the Sky and Dominating the Earth

Stand upright with the legs apart, rotate the palms upward, and move them to the sides. Lift the palms vigorously towards the sky first, and then towards the ground. Take a deep breath. Do the form again. (Figure 24.80)

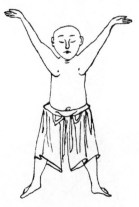

Figure 24.80

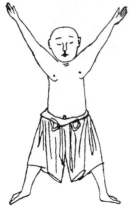

Figure 24.81

Coordination of the Four Limbs

Stand upright with the legs apart, push both hands to the sides, with the palms facing inwards, the left hand facing the right foot and vice-versa. Then, stretch the four limbs at the same time, and take a deep breath. Do the form again. (Figure 24.81)

Belfry

Stand upright with the legs apart, raise the hands over the head, with the palms together and the arms straight. Take three deep breaths. Do the form again. (Figure 24.82)

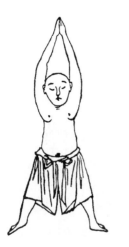

Figure 24.82

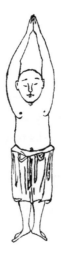

Figure 24.83

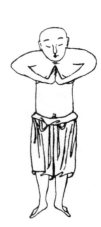

Figure 24.84

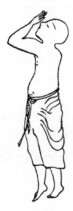

Figure 24.85

Standing Like a Pine

Stand with the feet together and the heels touching, and lift the soles off the ground. Stretch the body, and keep it as straight as a pine. Take three deep breaths. Do the form again. (Figure 24.83)

Returning to the "Presenting a Pestle" Form

From the final position in the last form, lower the soles of the feet and slowly lower the palms to shoulder level, being careful to keep them together at all times. Take three deep breaths. The rest are identical to the form with the same name on page 229. (Figure 24.84)

Turning the Face to the Sky

Identical to the form with the same name on page 230. (Figure 24.85)

Returning to the "Standing Straight with the Arms in an Arc" Form

Identical to the form with the same name on page 230. (Figure 24.86)

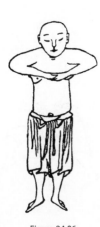

Figure 24.86

6. Exercises with the Body Turned

Presenting a Pestle on a Horse

Identical to the form with the same name on page 235. (Figure 24.87)

Turning the Body and Arms to the Left

Stand on the balls of the feet, turn the head and body to the left, bend the left knee and stretch the right leg, to form a semi-bow stance and with both feet perpendicular to each other. Keep the waist and head straight. Bring the hands together to the front of the nose. Keep the ears in line with the shoulders and the nose in line with the chest. Concentrate the mind, and look straight ahead. Take a deep breath. (Figure 24.88)

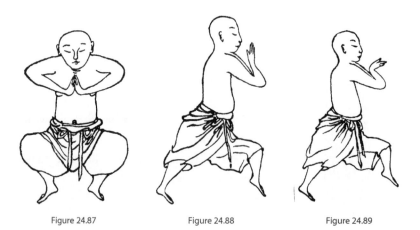

Figure 24.87   Figure 24.88   Figure 24.89

Turning the Body to the Left and Raising the Hands

Stand upright, hold the palms together and point them forward. Then return the hands to the sides and hold them as if they are holding heavy weights. Take a deep breath. Do the form again. (Figure 24.89)

Inclining to the Left

Open the palms at the sides of the body, raise them to touch the shoulders, and then press the palms down along the body, and place them flat on the ground. Fix the eyes on the ground. Make the mind a blank while you take three deep breaths. Do the form again. (Figure 24.90)

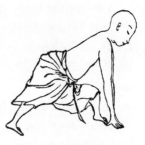

Figure 24.90

Returning to the Original Form on the Left

Rise slowly, and return to the "Turning the Body and Arms to the Left" form. Take a deep breath. Do the form again. (Figure 24.91)

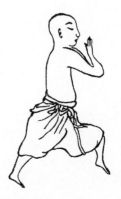

Figure 24.91

Turning the Body and Arms to the Right

This form is identical to "Turning the Body and Arms to the Left" on page 254, except that the movements are performed on the right. (Figure 24.92)

Turning the Body to the Right and Raising the Hands

This form is identical to "Turning the Body to the Left and Raising the Hands" on page 255, except that the movements are performed on the right. (Figure 24.93)

Inclining to the Right

This form is identical to "Inclining to the Left" on page 255, except that the movements are performed on the right. (Figure 24.94)

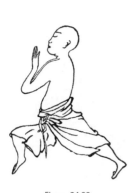
Figure 24.92

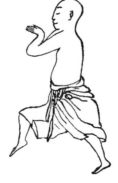
Figure 24.93

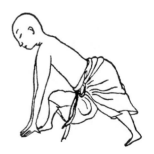
Figure 24.94

Returning to the Original Form on the Right

The movements are the same as for "Returning to the Original Form on the Left" on page 255, except performed in the opposite direction. (Figure 24.95)

Pulling the Ox's Tail to the Left

Clench the fists, turn the head and body to the left, and raise the left fist to the left until the left upper arm is in line with the left shoulder and the base of the left fist is facing the eyes. Lower the right hand while turning it towards the right thigh. Take three deep breaths. The stance is the same as in Figure 24.88. (Figure 24.96)

Pulling the Ox's Tail to the Right

The movements are the same as in the previous form, except performed in the opposite direction. (Figure 24.97)

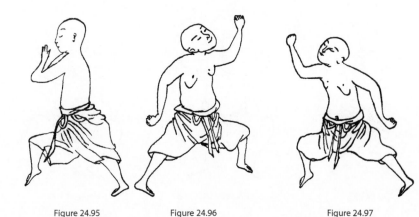

Figure 24.95   Figure 24.96   Figure 24.97

Presenting a Pestle with the Left Palm Erect

After the last form, draw the hands and feet back, and straighten the head and body. Balancing on the balls of the feet, adopt the horse-riding stance. Bend the left elbow, and keep the forearm level in front of the chest, with the left palm upright and facing the right. Bend the right elbow, and keep the right forearm level in front of the chest with the right palm facing down and under the left wrist. Take a deep breath. The other movements are identical to those of "Presenting a Pestle on a Horse" on page 235. (Figure 24.98)

Presenting a Pestle with the Right Palm Erect

The movements are the same as in the previous form, except performed in the opposite direction. (Figure 24.99)

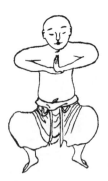
Figure 24.98

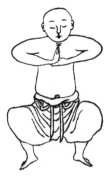
Figure 24.99

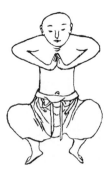
Figure 24.100

Presenting a Pestle and Returning to the Middle Form

Identical to the "Returning to the 'Presenting a Pestle on a Horse' Form" on page 243. (Figure 24.100)

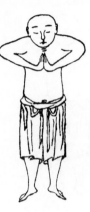

Rising in the Air

From the horse-riding stance, slowly raise the body, balancing on the balls of the feet, as if you are rising in the air. Take a deep breath. The other movements are the same as those for the "Returning to the 'Presenting a Pestle' Form" on page 229. (Figure 24.101)

Figure 24.101

Turning the Face to the Sky

Identical to the form with the same name on page 230. (Figure 24.102)

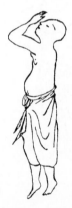

Figure 24.102

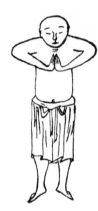

Figure 24.103

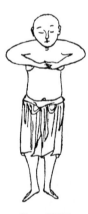

Figure 24.104

Returning to the "Presenting a Pestle" Form

Identical to the form with the same name on page 229. (Figure 24.103)

Returning to the "Standing Straight with the Arms in an Arc" Form

Identical to the form with the same name on page 230. (Figure 24.104)

7. Exercises in Crouching Positions
Presenting a Pestle on a Horse

Identical to the form with the same name on page 235. (Figure 24.105)

Holding the Palms Together Before the Chest

After the last form, draw the palms back close to the chest. Take three deep breaths, and then do the next form. Do this form again. (Figure 24.106)

On All Fours

After the last form, part the two palms, and hold them out at shoulder level. Lower them to the ground, with all ten fingers touching the ground. At the same time, raise the heels. Raise the head, and look up, with the eyes and mind focused. Take three deep breaths, starting with exhalation. Lead the *qi* to move in the reverse direction. See Chapter XIX for reference. Then do the next form. (Figure 24.107)

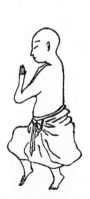

Figure 24.105

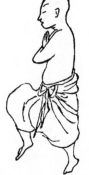

Figure 24.106

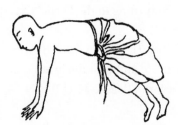

Figure 24.107

Tripod with the Left Foot

With the hands still placed on the ground, move the left foot forward, raise the heel, and lift the right foot behind until it is level with the head, back and buttocks, forming a tripod. Take three deep breaths, leading the *qi* to *niwan* (an acupuncture point in the head) and then to the heel. Repeat three times. (Figure 24.108)

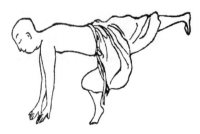

Figure 24.108

Tripod with the Right Foot

The movements are the same as in the previous form, except performed in the opposite direction. (Figure 24.109)

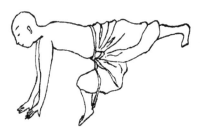

Figure 24.109

Returning to the Form "On All Fours"

Return to the "on all fours" position, and take the breaths as in that form. (Figure 24.110)

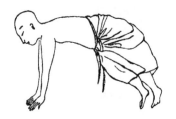

Figure 24.110

8. Exercises with the Body Turned Over

Sitting on the Ground

In the last position, move both feet forward to between the hands. Move the hands to the outer sides of the thighs. Then lift the heels off the ground, and make them touch to form a "V." Keep the head and body upright, and look straight ahead. Concentrate the mind and take three deep breaths. (Figure 24.111)

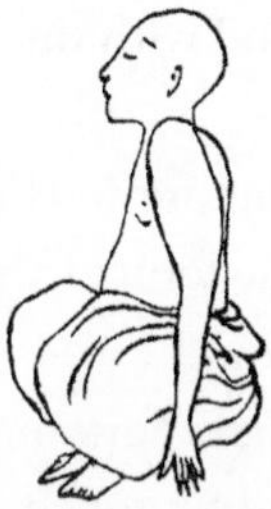

Figure 24.111

Turning the Body Over

Extend the feet forwards and the hands backwards. Support the body with the fingers and toes. The body should be horizontal. Take three deep breaths, and lead the *qi* in a reverse direction. (Figure 24.112)

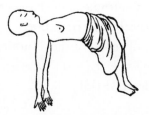

Figure 24.112

Tripod with the Left Foot in the Air

In the previous position, move the right foot to the central-back position, the toes touching the ground and forming a tripod with the handing touching the ground supporting the body. Raise the left foot and stretch it forward as far as possible. Fix the gaze on the left instep. Take three deep breaths. (Figure 24.113)

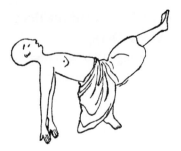

Figure 24.113

Tripod with the Right Foot in the Air

Same as the last form, except that you raise the right foot. (Figure 24.114)

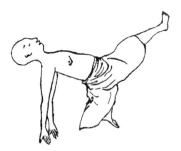

Figure 24.114

Returning to the Form of "Turning the Body Over"

Identical to the "Turning the Body Over" form on page 263. (Figure 24.115)

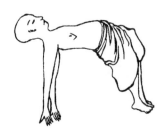

Figure 24.115

Holding the Palms Together In Front of the Chest

Draw the feet back and stand erect. Lift the heels off the ground so that just the toes touch the ground. Bend the legs and knees, keeping the body upright. Hold the palms together before the chest with eyes looking forward. Take three deep breaths and then do the next form. (Figure 24.116)

Saluting High on a Horse

After the last form, keep the toes on the ground. Keep the palms together and move them up and stretch as if saluting on a horse. Take a deep breath, lead the *qi* up. Then quickly go to the next form. (Figure 24.117)

Saluting Low on a Horse

Balanced on the balls of both feet, squat and touch the ground with the tips of the fingers of both hands, and with the palms together. Keep the eyes focused to the front. Take a deep breath, and lead the *qi* down. (Figure 24.118)

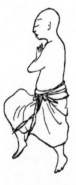 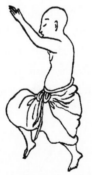 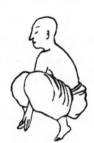

Figure 24.116   Figure 24.117   Figure 24.118

Three Rises and Falls

Stand on the balls of the feet. Hold the palms together as in the "Presenting a Pestle" form on page 220. Take a deep breath, keeping the spine upright and the knees bent. Squat and lower the hands until the upper arms are between the knees. Rise, keeping the palms together. Repeat the movements three times. With every rise and fall, take a deep breath and draw the palms back a bit closer to the chest until they touch the chest. Repeat the rise and fall once more before going on to the next form. (Figure 24.119)

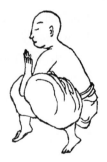

Figure 24.119

Standing Straight with Three Pushes

Stand on the balls of the feet. Keep the body upright, and hold the palms together close to the chest. Take a deep breath. Then push the palms out, and take another deep breath. Push three times in total, then return to the "Presenting a Pestle" form on page 220. Take another deep breath, and lower the heels to the ground. (Figure 24.120)

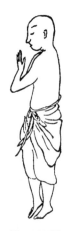

Figure 24.120

Turning the Face to the Sky

Identical to the form of the same name on page 230. (Figure 24.121)

Returning to the "Presenting a Pestle" Form

Identical to the form of the same name on page 253. (Figure 24.122)

Returning to the "Standing Straight with the Arms in an Arc" Form

Identical to the form of the same name on page 253. (Figure 24.123)

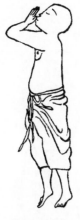
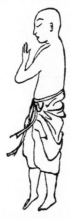
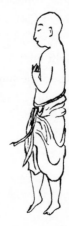

Figure 24.121   Figure 24.122   Figure 24.123

9. EXERCISES IN A MARCHING POSITION
Left Foot

Keep the body and head upright, and eyes looking forward. Stretch the arms with the fingers interlaced and the palms facing down. Root the right foot firmly on the ground. Bend the left knee, lift it across to the right side, and then kick hard with the left foot to the left. Take a deep breath. Note that when practicing this form you should only move the left leg and not any other part of the body. Kick 45 times in a row, each time accompanied by a deep breath. (Figure 24.124)

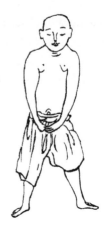

Figure 24.124

Right Foot

Repeat the above movements with the right foot. (Figure 24.125)

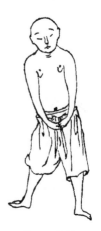

Figure 24.125

Right Foot Kick to the Front

Keep the left foot firmly on the ground. Lift the right foot and move it to above the instep of the left foot. Then kick the right foot towards the front once without moving any other part of the body. Take a deep breath. Kick 36 times in a row, each time accompanied by a deep breath. (Figure 24.126)

Left Foot Kick to the Front

The same as the last form, except using the left foot. Together with the 45 kicks mentioned before, each foot kicks 81 times. (Figure 24.127)

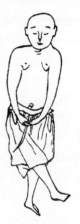

Figure 24.126

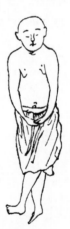

Figure 24.127

Lowering the Palms and Pounding the Ground

Move the heels close to each other, and interlace the fingers. Turn the palms towards the sky, and then lower them to the level of the toes. Lift the heels, and lower them to pound the ground. Take a deep breath. Repeat these movements 21 times. Keep the body straight and eyes looking straight ahead. (Figure 24.128)

Relaxing the Brows Form 1

Cross the wrists, with the palms facing outwards. Raise the hands to between the brows. Touch the right brow with the left hand, and the left brow with the right hand. Take a deep breath. (Figure 24.129)

Relaxing the Brows Form 2

Separate the crossed hands, and stretch the arms fully to their respective sides. Take a deep breath. (Figure 24.130)

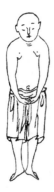

Figure 24.128

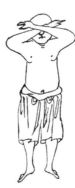

Figure 24.129

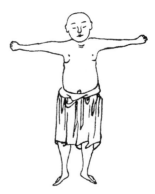

Figure 24.130

Relaxing the Brows Form 3

Straighten the spine, and bend the knees to squat, with the heels firmly planted on the ground and the balls of the feet raised. Fold the arms, and place them against the brows. Push the elbows with force to the left and right, respectively. Take a deep breath. (Figure 24.131)

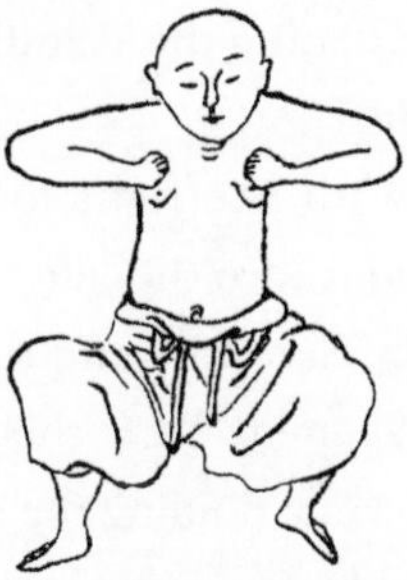

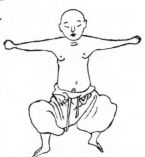

Figure 24.131

Relaxing the Brows Form 4

Still in the squatting position, clench the fists and stretch the arms forcefully to their respective sides. Take a deep breath. (Figure 24.132)

The above four forms should be practiced three times to complete the set of movements.

Figure 24.132

Turning the Windlass to the Left
Form 1
With the right foot pointing diagonally ahead, move the left foot forward so the sole of the right foot and the tiptoe of the left foot are aligned. Turn the head and body to the left, while holding the arms straight in front at shoulder height and the palms downward. Take a deep breath. (Figure 24.133)

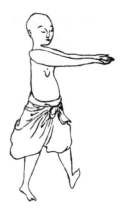

Figure 24.133

Turning the Windlass to the Left
Form 2
With the arms stretched as in the last form, turn the palms upward, and clench the fists. Turn the fists downward, and swing the arms down to the outer sides of the thighs. Take a deep breath. (Figure 24.134)

Turning the Windlass to the Left
Form 3
Turn the backs of the fists to face the ground. Bend the elbows, with the upper arms pressed against the armpits, until the arms form a 90-degree angle. Take a deep breath. (Figure 24.135)

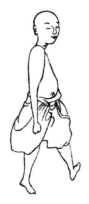

Figure 24.134

Turning the Windlass to the Left Form 4

Draw the left foot back and put it behind the right foot, with the left toes touching the ground. Rotate the fists inwards, and let them hang down as you lower your body. Take a deep breath. (Figure 24.136)

Turning the Windlass to the Left Form 5

Stand firm with the heels together and the toes facing outwards. Straighten the body, allowing the arms to hang down, with the fists clenched at the sides. Take a deep breath. (Figure 24.137)

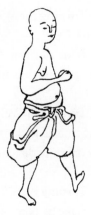

Figure 24.135

Turning the Windlass to the Right Form 1

Same as Form 1 on page 272, but done in the opposite direction. (Figure 24.138)

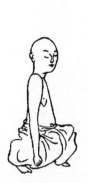

Figure 24.136

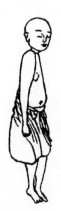

Figure 24.137

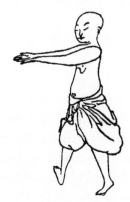

Figure 24.138

Turning the Windlass to the Right
Form 2

Same as Form 2 on page 272, but done in the opposite direction. (Figure 24.139)

Turning the Windlass to the Right Form 3

Same as Form 3 on page 272, but done in the opposite direction. (Figure 24.140)

Turning the Windlass to the Right Form 4

Same as Form 4 on page 273, but done in the opposite direction. (Figure 24.141)

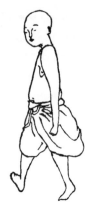

Figure 24.139

Turning the Windlass to the Right Form 5

Same as Form 5 on page 273, but done in the opposite direction. (Figure 24.142)

Note

There are two ways to practice the "Turning the Windlass" forms: turning the windlass to the left and then to the right is called "Single Windlass"; to practice the forms on both sides separately is called "Double Windlass." The practice described in this book is the "Single Windlass," which needs to be done three times each session.

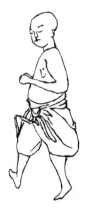

Figure 24.140

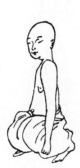

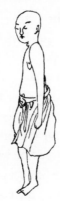

Figure 24.141   Figure 24.142

Rising in the Air on the Left

Place both feet firmly on the ground, the spine straight, the fists clenched and the arms hanging naturally. Keep the ears directly above the shoulders and the tip of the nose vertically in line with the chest, eyes looking straight ahead, teeth clenched and the tip of the tongue touching the upper palate. Take three deep breaths, then lift up the left foot and take one step forward. Stretch the left leg, and take a deep breath. (Figure 24.143)

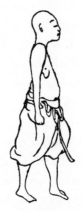

Figure 24.143

Rising in the Air on the Right

Same as the last form, but done in the opposite direction. (Figure 24.144)

The two above forms together are called the "Diagram of the Sun and Moon" or the "Diagram of Taiji." Breath control and mental concentration are the same as for the other forms. The eyes can be either closed or wide open, but they should always be fixed on a spot between 33 cm and 1.6 m away from the body.

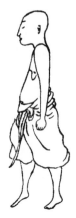

Figure 24.144

The Superior Aureole

In this form, the stance is the same as in the form "Standing Straight with the Arms held in an Arc" on page 219, except that the arms dangle loosely by the sides, with the fists clenched. After the breath has been calmed, cross the arms below the navel, and move them up to cross above the head. Take a deep breath. (Figure 24.145)

The Inferior Aureole

After the last form, move the crossed hands down to below the navel, with the hands still crossed. Take a deep breath. Practice the "Small Heavenly Circulation" of qi three times, and

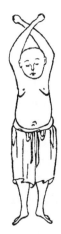

Figure 24.145

then take three deep breaths. Separate the hands, and let them hang naturally. (Figure 24.146)

The Fish Flaps its Fins at the Back

Clench the fists, and swing the arms from the sides to the rear. Take a deep breath. (Figure 24.147)

The Fish Flaps its Fins at the Front

From the previous position, swing the arms to the front, making them pass close to the sides of the body. Then, with the backs of the fists facing the front, separate the fists and move them to the sides. Take a deep breath. (Figure 24.148)

This exercise is completed by repeating the previous two forms three times.

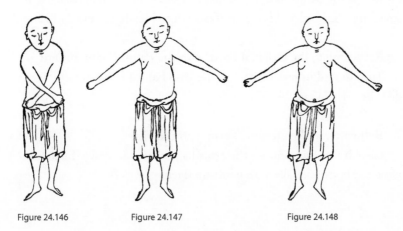

Figure 24.146   Figure 24.147   Figure 24.148

The Fish Flaps its Fins on its Back
In the final position of the last form, pound the back of the body with the fists, arms always kept straight. Take a deep breath. (Figure 24.149)

The Fish Flaps its Fins on its Front
Push the fists towards the front, brushing the sides of the body, arms always kept straight. Inhale, and repeat this movement three times, exhaling and inhaling each time. (Figure 24.150)

Returning to the Original Form with the Palms
Let the arms dangle, unclench the fists, while stretching the head and body up. Take a deep breath. (Figure 24.151)

Returning to the Original Form with the Backs of the Hands
Rotate the palms so that the backs of the hands face outward, while stretching the head and body up. Take a deep breath. (Figure 24.152)

Returning to the Original Form with the Palms Facing Inward
Turn the palms inward, and let the arms hang down naturally. Take a deep breath. (Figure 24.153)

Returning to the Original Form with the Fists
Clench the fists, and let the arms hang down naturally. Stretch the neck and body up. Take a deep breath. (Figure 24.154)

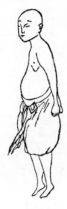

Figure 24.149

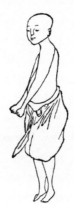

Figure 24.150

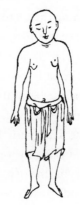

Figure 24.151

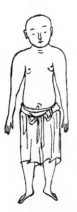

Figure 24.152

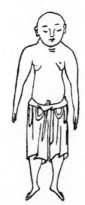

Figure 24.153

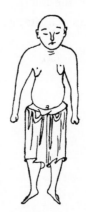

Figure 24.154

Leading the *Qi* to the Origin

Loosen the fists, and place the right palm on *huangting* (in the center of the breast) and the left palm below the navel. Push the right palm down to below the navel while pushing the left palm up along the left side of the body to *huangting*. Then push the left palm back to below the navel along the original route, at the same time moving the right palm along the right side of the body. Take a deep breath. After finishing the pushing movement with both hands, repeat the movement 21 times, taking deep breaths 21 times. In this way, the *qi* will return to the *dantian* and the mind will be concentrated to nourish the internal organs later during the Exercises in a Sitting Position. (Figure 24.155)

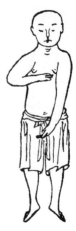

Figure 24.155

Returning to the Original Form with the Hands on the Hips

Place the hands on the hips, with the thumbs facing forwards and the fingers facing backwards. Take a deep breath. (Figure 24.156)

Returning to the Form of the Arms in an Arc

Draw both hands back to return to the form of the arms in an arc. Take three deep breaths, each time hurriedly at the beginning and slowly at the end. Calm the self and focus the attention on *qihai* (about 6.6 cm below the navel).

This is the end of the Exercises in a Marching Position. (Figure 24.157)

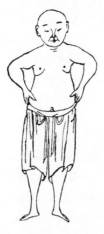

Figure 24.156

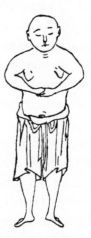

Figure 24.157

10. Exercises in a Sitting Position

Concentrating the Attention on One Fist

In a seated position, place the left foot on the right thigh and the right foot on the left thigh. Hold the left arm level across the chest, palm facing up. Clench the right fist and place it on the left palm. Straighten the back, eyes looking straight ahead. Keep the ears vertically in line with the shoulders and the nose in line with the chest. The teeth should be clenched and the tongue touching the upper palate. Breathe following the rhythm of the "Small Heavenly Circulation" of *qi*. When exhaling, lower the *qi* to the *dantian*; when inhaling, lead the *qi* up *dumai* (Governing Meridian). Practice the circulation of *qi* three times.

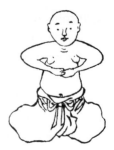

Figure 24.158

The previous forms teach the methods of the production of *qi*, while this one shows how to conduct the *qi* to the spirit. (Figure 24.158)

Sitting with the Palms Held Together

Sit as in the previous form. The movements of the upper body are the same as in "Presenting a Pestle" (see Figure 24.2) in the first part. Take three deep breaths so as to concentrate the *qi* in the internal organs. (Figure 24.159)

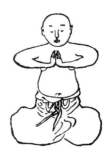

Figure 24.159

Pushing the Door with Both Hands

Sit as in the previous form. The movements of the upper body are the same as in "Producing the Claws and Displaying the Wings" on page 220. Push both arms straight forward level with the shoulders and with the palms erect and facing outwards. Take three deep breaths so as to move the *qi* to all the meridians of the body. (Figure 24.160)

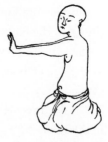

Figure 24.160

Harmonizing the *Qi*

Sit as in the previous form. The movements of the upper body resemble the "Double Phoenixes Salute the Sun" form on page 221. Take three deep breaths so as to activate and harmonize the *qi*. (Figure 24.161)

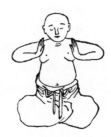

Figure 24.161

Extending the Arms and Regulating the *Qi* in the Meridians

Sit as in the previous form. The movements of the upper body resemble "The Eagle Spreading its Wings" form on page 221. Take three deep breaths, extend the arms and regulate the *qi* in all the meridians. (Figure 24.162)

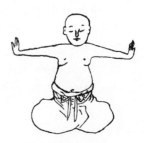

Figure 24.162

Supporting Emptiness and Smoothing the *Qi* in the Stomach

Sit as in the previous form. The movements of the upper body are the same as those in "Supporting a Tower with Both Hands" on page 222. Take three deep breaths to smooth the *qi* in the stomach. (Figure 24.163)

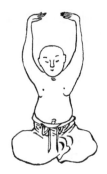

Figure 24.163

Supporting Burdens with the Arms Close to the Armpits

Sit as in the previous form. The movements of the upper body resemble the "Three Peaks" form on page 222. Take three deep breaths, and press the arms closely against the armpits. (Figure 24.164)

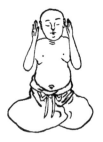

Figure 24.164

Dispersing Negative Energy in the Liver and Lungs on the Left

Sit as in the previous form. The movements of the upper body are the same as those in "The Dragon Sticking out its Right Claw" on page 223. Take three deep breaths to regulate the circulation of *qi* in the lungs. (Figure 24.165)

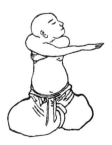

Figure 24.165

Dispersing Negative Energy in the Liver and Lungs on the Right

Sit as in the previous form. The movements of the upper body are the same as those in "The Dragon Sticking out its Left Claw" on page 223. Take three deep breaths to regulate the circulation of *qi* in the liver. (Figure 24.166)

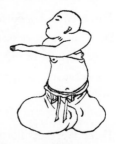

Figure 24.166

Sitting with the Arms Held Horizontally

Sit as in the previous form. The movements of the upper body are the same as those in "Squatting with Arms Held Horizontally" on page 224. Take three deep breaths to make the *qi* circulate in the limbs. (Figure 24.167)

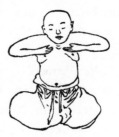

Figure 24.167

Three Warmers Form 1

Sit as in the previous form. The movements of the upper body are the same as those in the "Circulation of *Qi* Form 1" on page 224. Take a deep breath to concentrate the *qi* at *shangjiao* (Upper Warmer, the cavity above the diaphragm). (Figure 24.168)

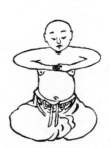

Figure 24.168

Three Warmers Form 2

Sit as in the previous form. The movements of the upper body are the same as those in the "Circulation of *Qi* Form 2" on page 224. Take a deep breath to concentrate the *qi* at *xiajiao* (Lower Warmer, the abdomen). (Figure 24.169)

Three Warmers Form 3

Sit as in the previous form. The movements of the upper body are the same as those in the "Circulation of *Qi* Form 3" on page 225. Take a deep breath to concentrate the *qi* at *zhongjiao* (Middle Warmer, around the navel). (Figure 24.170)

Three Warmers Form 4

Sit as in the previous form. The movements of the upper body are the same as those in the "Circulation of *Qi* Form 4" on page 225. Take a deep breath to smooth *zhongjiao*. (Figure 24.171)

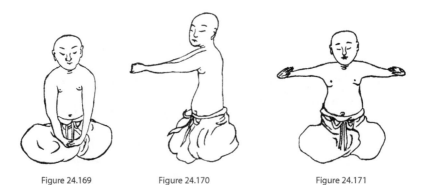

Figure 24.169   Figure 24.170   Figure 24.171

Three Warmers Form 5

Sit as in the previous form. The movements of the upper body resemble the "Circulation of *Qi* Form 5" on page 226. Take a deep breath to make the *qi* descend from *zhongjiao* to *xiajiao*. (Figure 24.172)

Three Warmers Form 6

Sit as in the previous form. The movements of the upper body are the same as those in the "Circulation of *Qi* Form 6" on page 226. Take a deep breath to move the *qi* from *xiajiao* to *zhongjiao*. (Figure 24.173)

Three Warmers Form 7

Sit as in the previous form. The movements of the upper body are the same as those in the "Circulation of *Qi* Form 7" on page 227. Take a deep breath to fill *zhongjiao* with *qi*. (Figure 24.174)

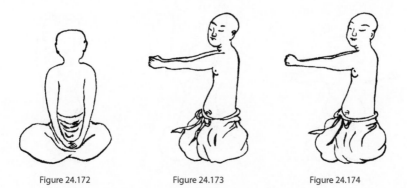

Figure 24.172   Figure 24.173   Figure 24.174

Three Warmers Form 8

Sit as in the previous form. The movements of the upper body are the same as those in the "Circulation of *Qi* Form 8" on page 227. Take a deep breath to disperse the *qi* in *zhongjiao*. (Figure 24.175)

Three Warmers Form 9

Sit as in the previous form. The movements of the upper body are the same as those in the "Circulation of *Qi* Form 9" on page 227. Take a deep breath to make the *qi* circulate from *zhongjiao* to *shangjiao*. (Figure 24.176)

Three Warmers Form 10

Sit as in the previous form. The movements of the upper body are the same as those in the "Circulation of *Qi* Form 10" on page 228. Take a deep breath so that light and pure *qi* diffuses at *shangjiao*. (Figure 24.177)

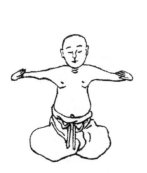
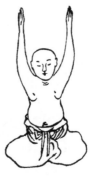
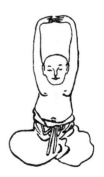

Figure 24.175   Figure 24.176   Figure 24.177

Three Warmers Form 11

Sit as in the previous form. The movements of the upper body are the same as those in the "Circulation of Qi Form 11" on page 228. Take a deep breath to return the *qi* of pure *yang* to *zhongjiao*. (Figure 24.178)

Three Warmers Form 12

Sit as in the previous form. The movements of the upper body are the same as those in the "Circulation of Qi Form 12" on page 228. Take a deep breath to fill *zhongjiao* with the *qi* of pure *yang*. (Figure 24.179)

Three Warmers Form 13

Sit as in the previous form. The movements of the upper body are the same as those in the "Circulation of Qi Form 13" on page 228. Take a deep breath to disperse the *qi* of pure *yang* in *zhongjiao*. (Figure 24.180)

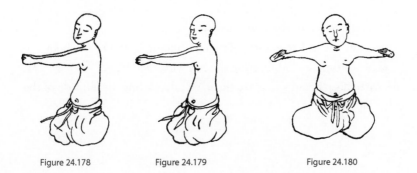

Figure 24.178   Figure 24.179   Figure 24.180

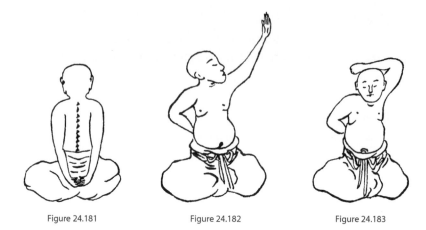

Figure 24.181   Figure 24.182   Figure 24.183

Three Warmers Form 14

Sit as in the previous form. The movements of the upper body are the same as in the "Circulation of *Qi* Form 14" on page 229. Take a deep breath to make the heavy and turbid *qi* descend to *xiajiao*. (Figure 24.181)

Plucking Stars on the Left Form 1

Sit as in the previous form. The movements of the upper body are the same as those in "Supporting the Sky with One Hand" on page 231. Take three deep breaths to make the *qi* circulate along the left side of the body. (Figure 24.182)

Plucking Stars on the Left Form 2

Sit as in the previous form. The movements of the upper body are the same as those in the "Drawing a Sword While Turning the Hand" form on page 231. Take three breaths to make the *qi* circulate along the right side of the body. (Figure 24.183)

Plucking Stars on the Left Form 3

Sit as in the previous form. The movements of the upper body are the same as those in "Drawing the Bow" on page 232. Take three deep breaths to harmonize the *qi* in the liver. (Figure 24.184)

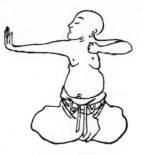

Figure 24.184

Plucking Stars on the Right Form 1

Identical to "Plucking Stars on the Left Form 1" on page 290, except in the opposite direction. Take three deep breaths to direct the *qi* to the right. (Figure 24.185)

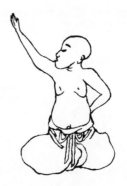

Figure 24.185

Plucking Stars on the Right Form 2

Identical to "Plucking Stars on the Left Form 2" on page 291, except in the opposite direction. Take three deep breaths to make the *qi* circulate along the left side of the body. (Figure 24.186)

Plucking Stars on the Right Form 3

Identical to "Plucking Stars on the Left Form 3" on page 291, except in the opposite direction. Take three deep breaths to moisturize the lungs with *qi*. (Figure 24.187)

These are the six forms of "Plucking Stars." They promote the circulation of *qi*. The pure *qi* floats to the top of the head.

Keeping the Arms Level, Palms Facing Down

Sit as in the previous form. Extend the arms to the front, level with the shoulders and with the palms facing downwards. Move the arms to the right and left, respectively until they are horizontal. Take a deep breath to smooth *zhongjiao* with *qi*. (Figure 24.188)

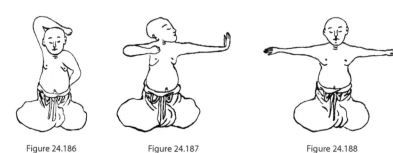

Figure 24.186   Figure 24.187   Figure 24.188

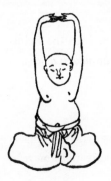

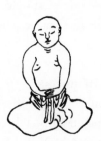

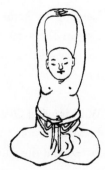

Figure 24.189   Figure 24.190   Figure 24.191

Supporting the Void with Both Hands

Sit as in the previous form. Raise the arms above the head. Make the fingertips touch, with the palms facing upwards. Take a deep breath to smooth *shangjiao* with *qi*. (Figure 24.189)

Calming the Spirit and Making Qi Descend

Sit as in the previous form. Lower the hands to the thighs, with the fingers interlaced. Calm the spirit, take a deep breath, and make *qi* descend from *shangjiao* to *xiajiao*. (Figure 24.190)

Support the Void Again with Both Hands

Raise the arms above the head again, palms facing up. Take a deep breath to send *qi* to *shangjiao*. (Figure 24.191)

Keeping the Arms Level, Palms Facing Up

Extend the arms to either side at shoulder level, with the palms turned upwards. Take a deep breath to move *qi* from *shangjiao* to *zhongjiao*. (Figure 24.192)

Withdrawing *Qi* and the Palms

Lower the arms from shoulder level to the thighs, with the fingers interlaced and the palms facing upwards. Take a deep breath to move *qi* from *zhongjiao* to *xiajiao*. (Figure 24.193)

Returning to the Form "Keeping the Arms Level, Palms Facing Down"

Stretch the arms out sideways at shoulder level, with the palms turned down. Take a deep breath to move *qi* from *xiajiao* to *zhongjiao*. (Figure 24.194)

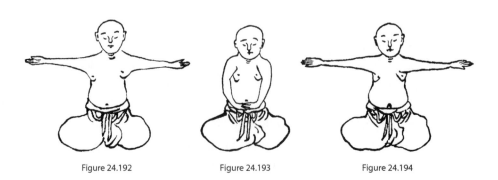

Figure 24.192   Figure 24.193   Figure 24.194

Returning to the Form "Withdrawing *Qi* and the Palms"

This form is identical to "Withdrawing *Qi* and the Palms" on page 294. Repeat the movement slowly three times. Every time breathe deeply in and out once to make the *qi* of the three *jiao* (*shangjiao*, *zhongjiao* and *xiajiao*) return to its original places. (Figure 24.195)

The Cross Form, Hands Down at the Lower Body

Extend the arms forward and cross them close to and in front of the body, palms facing down. Then separate the arms, and extend them to either side at shoulder level. Take a deep breath to smooth *qi* throughout the body. (Figure 24.196)

The Cross Form, Palms Facing Down

Raise the arms to shoulder level, and stretch them horizontally to either side. Take a deep breath to make *qi* circulate throughout the body. (Figure 24.197)

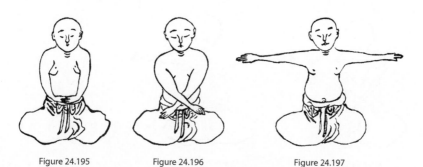

Figure 24.195   Figure 24.196   Figure 24.197

The Cross Form, Withdrawing the Palms

Lower the arms to the sides, then cross them in front of the body. Make the hands touch the opposite shoulders. Concentrate the attention at the point of *qihai* (about 6.6 cm below the navel). Take a deep breath to make *qi* circulate throughout the meridians. (Figure 24.198)

The Cross Form, Palms Facing Up

Cross the arms in front of the chest, palms facing up. Then stretch the arms horizontally to the sides at shoulder level and with the palms facing upwards. Take a deep breath to make *qi* circulate throughout the body. Turn the palms to face downwards. Take a deep breath to unblock the *qi* in the meridians. (Figure 24.199)

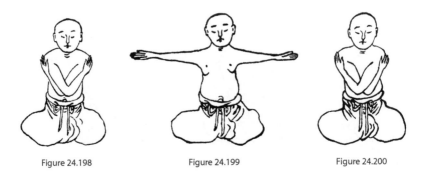

Figure 24.198   Figure 24.199   Figure 24.200

The Cross Form, Holding the Shoulders

Cross the palms in front of the body, touching the chest. Extend the hands to touch the opposite shoulders. Keep the elbows down. Concentrate the attention at *qihai* (6.6 cm below the navel). Take a deep breath to make the *qi* circulate throughout the body. (Figure 24.200)

The Cross Form, Returning to the "Palms Facing Down" Form

Cross the arms in front of the body at shoulder level, palms facing down. Straighten the spine, then stretch the arms out horizontally to each side. Take a deep breath to make the *qi* circulate freely upwards and downwards. (Figure 24.201)

The Cross Form, Clenching the Fists

With the arms stretched out to the sides at shoulder level, clench the fists. Take a deep breath to block all the orifices of the body. (Figure 24.202)

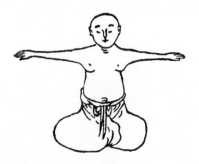

Figure 24.201

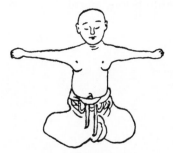

Figure 24.202

The Cross Form, Withdrawing the Fists

Draw the fists back towards the shoulders, and then place them on the hips. Take a deep breath to block all the orifices of the body. (Figure 24.203)

The Cross Form, Hands on Hips

Unclench the fists, leaving the hands on the hips, with the thumbs pointing forwards and the fingers pointing to the rear. Take a deep breath to block all the orifices of the body. (Figure 24.204)

Overlapping the Hands

Place the hands overlapping each other on the crossed legs. Calm the mind and *qi*. (Figure 24.205)

Returning to the "Concentrating the Attention on One Fist" Form

Sit as the previous form. Clench the right fist and hold it with the left palm to form a circle with the arms in front of the chest. Take three deep breaths before returning to the first form on page 282. (Figure 24.206)

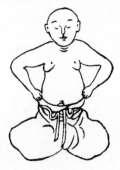

Figure 24.203

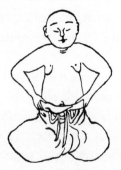

Figure 24.204

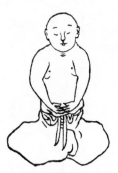

Figure 24.205

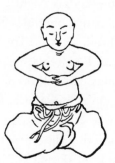

Figure 24.206

11. Exercises with the Body Upright
Calming the *Qi* and Harmonizing the Spirit

This form is identical to the first form in the last section on page 282, except that the orifices and vital points are closed to calm the *qi*. In addition, the eyes should focus on the interior of the body to harmonize the spirit. Inhale to make *qi* descend, and exhale to make it ascend. Exhale and inhale three times. (Figure 24.207)

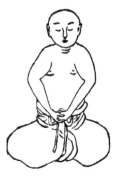

Figure 24.207

The Cycle of the Sun and Moon

Sit with the body straight and the legs crossed, and holding one fist with the palm of the other hand, as in the last form. *Qihai* is slightly closed. Revolve the eyeballs counterclockwise 21 times. Take 21 deep breaths, and swallow the saliva three times. Revolve the eyeballs clockwise 21 times, and take 21 deep breaths. Swallow the saliva three times before doing the next form. (Figure 24.208)

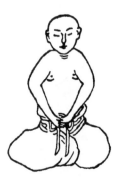

Figure 24.208

Remounting to the Clear Source

Sit with the legs crossed, keeping the spine straight, and with the tip of the tongue touching the upper palate and the eyes gazing straight ahead. Hold the left fist with the right palm, and place them on the crossed legs. Take three deep breaths. Make *qi* descend when inhaling, and ascend when exhaling. The *qi* should circulate in an inverse direction along the "Small Heavenly Circulation." (Figure 24.209)

Focusing on the Interior of the Body

Sit with the body erect, legs crossed and the left fist held in the right palm. Take three deep breaths. When inhaling, focus the eyes on the nose, and visualize the heart and kidneys in the mind. When exhaling, lead the *qi* inversely along the "Small Heavenly Circulation." When practicing this form, do not neglect nor rush to complete the circulation of the *qi*. In the first case, the *qi* will not reach its destination; in the second case, the *qi* will stagnate in the body. If the *qi* circulates at a moderate speed it can invigorate the internal organs. (Figure 24.210)

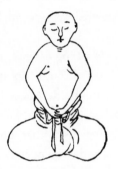

Figure 24.209

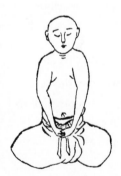

Figure 24.210

Marching Dragons and Tigers

In this form, the body position is the same as for the last form, with the teeth clenched and the tongue touching the upper palate. Take 21 deep, slow breaths. Swallow the saliva three times after every seventh breath. (Figure 24.211)

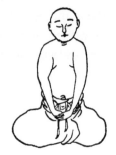

Figure 24.211

Absorbing Essence to Favor the Spirit

Sit with both legs stretched forward and the palms on the knees. Make *qi* descend when inhaling, and ascend when exhaling. Take three deep breaths so that the essence of the saliva, blood and *qi* can nurture the brain and enhance the intelligence. (Figure 24.212)

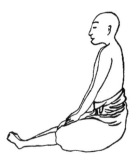

Figure 24.212

Returning to the Original Position

Bend the elbows, draw both legs back and bring the soles of the feet together. Straighten the arms, with the palms held together and the fingers interlaced and holding the toes together. Slowly breathe seven times, and swallow the saliva three times to concentrate the vital energy and return it to its original position. (Figure 24.213)

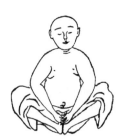

Figure 24.213

Nourishing the Vital Energy and Returning it to its Origin

Sit in the first position described on page 282. Weaken the respiration until the breath cannot be heard or felt any more. Only the vital energy is still active and abundant. (Figure 24.214)

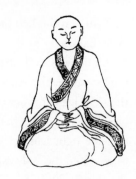

Figure 24.214

12. RECUMBENT EXERCISES
On the Left Side

Lie on the left side, with the left knee bent and the right leg stretched out. Hold the right shoulder with the left hand, and press the right hand on the floor in front of you. (Figure 24.215)

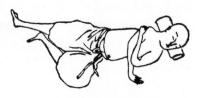

Figure 24. 215

On the Right Side

Same as the previous form, except done on the opposite side. (Figure 24.216)

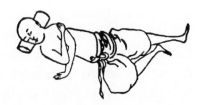

Figure 24.216

Lying on the Left Side with the Belly Exposed

Lie down with the head turned to the left, the left leg stretched out and the right leg bent. Let the left hand lie on the floor with the palm facing up. The right hand clasps the right thigh. Keep the belly exposed to the sky. (Figure 24.217)

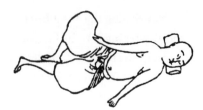

Figure 24.217

Lying on the Right Side with the Belly Exposed

Same as the previous form, except done on the opposite side. (Figure 24.218)

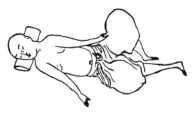

Figure 24.218

Lying on the Left Side with the Legs Bent

Lie down with the head turned to the left, the left knee raised and the left foot on the ground. The right leg should be bent and lying flat. Rest the left hand on the ground, palm facing up, and press the right hand on the right thigh. Keep the belly exposed to the sky. (Figure 24.219)

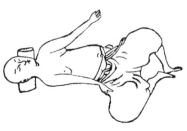

Figure 24.219

Lying on the Right Side with the Legs Bent

Same as the previous form, except done on the opposite side. (Figure 24.220)

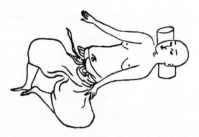

Figure 24.220

Lying on the Left Side and Arching the Body

Lie down with the head turned to the left and both legs bent. Place the right leg on the left one. Adjust the penis and scrotum to prevent the inner sides of the thighs touching each other. Hold the right shoulder with the left hand, and press the right hand on the floor. Arch the back. (Figure 24.221)

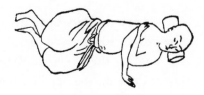

Figure 24.221

Lying on the Right Side and Arching the Body

Same as the previous form, except done on the opposite side. (Figure 24.222)

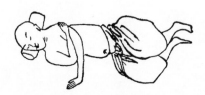

Figure 24.222

Lying on the Back and a Bit Towards the Left

Lie down with the head slightly turned to the left and the belly exposed. Place the left foot on the right one and the fists on the thighs. This form is used particularly when the circulation of *qi* in the left side of the body is not smooth. (Figure 24.223)

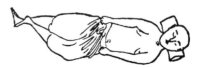

Figure 24.223

Lying on the Back and a Bit Towards the Right

Same as the previous form, except done on the opposite side. (Figure 24.224)

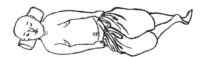

Figure 24.224

XXV

Twelve Massage Methods

The illustrations of Twelve Massage Methods were recorded in the book *Secret Methods of Massage and Daoyin Health Preservation*, by an anonymous author. The book contains 12 colorful ink paintings. Here we reproduce these paintings according to the Yunping version.

Method for Calming the Lungs and Dispelling Internal Heat

Application: Cough.

Method: Lie down on one side, put both hands under the neck, and bend both legs until the knees are higher than the abdomen. This position helps to dispel internal heat from the heart. If the internal heat in the heart stops affecting the lungs, the spirit will recover, and the cough will be cured. (Figure 25.1)

Method for Boosting the Spirit

Application: Neurasthenia.

Method: Lie down on the back, hold both knees with both hands as close to the body as possible. This position can help to produce strength, boost the spirit, dispel diseases and prolong life. (Figure 25.2)

Method of Circulating Qi

Application: Stagnation of *qi* in the lungs.

Method: Squat with both hands on the knees and lean back as far as you can, until you feel the resonance of the three *jiao* (Visceral Cavities). (Figure 25.3)

Method for Eliminating Stagnation and Indigestion

Application: Stagnation of *qi* and indigestion.

Method: Stand straight. Bend one elbow and stretch the other arm out to the side. Alternate the positions of the arms. After a while, hold the breath and click the teeth until all the air in the lungs is used up. (Figure 25.4)

Beating the Celestial Drum

Application: Dizziness and vision problems caused by external factors of cold or internal heat in the liver and stomach.

Method: Squat, cover the ears with the hands and at the same time tap the back of the head 49 times with the fingers while clicking the teeth 49 times. (Figure 25.5)

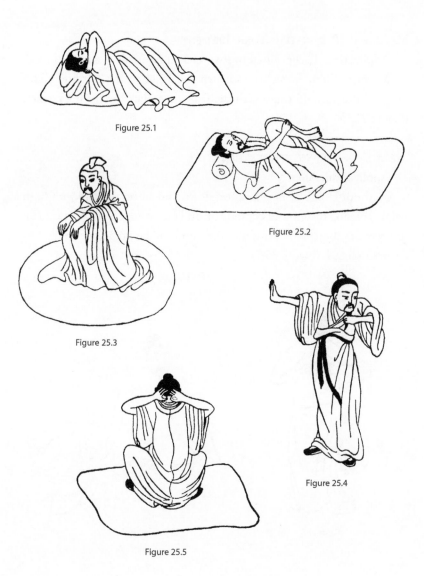

Figure 25.1

Figure 25.2

Figure 25.3

Figure 25.4

Figure 25.5

METHOD OF ELIMINATING TOXIC ELEMENTS

Application: Ulcer caused by toxic elements circulating in the blood.

Method: Stand straight, and turn the head to the left and right. Pummel the back 45 times with the fists, then click the teeth 45 times. (Figure 25.6)

METHOD OF STRENGTHENING THE HEART

Application: Anxiety.

Method: Hold the breath, kneel down and sit on the legs with both palms pressing the ground behind you and eyes wide open. Get rid of all unnecessary thoughts. In this way, the mind will be calmed naturally and desires reduced. (Figure 25.7)

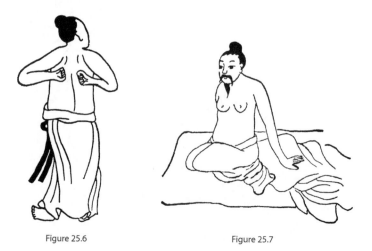

Figure 25.6   Figure 25.7

METHOD OF REGULATING THE FUNCTIONS OF THE KIDNEYS

Application: Pain in the kidneys or hernia.

Method: Stand straight, slowly warm the kidneys through massaging the back of the waist until you feel that it is burning hot. Then press the painful spots with the fingers to guide *qi* into them. In this way, the kidney pain can be stopped and the hernia treated. (Figure 25.8)

METHOD OF STIMULATING THE BLOOD CIRCULATION

Application: Rheumatic pain.

Method: Sit with the legs bent. Hold one foot with both hands, and lift it up as high as possible. Repeat with alternate feet until the four limbs perspire. In this way, *qi* and blood are harmonized and rheumatic pain treated. (Figure 25.9)

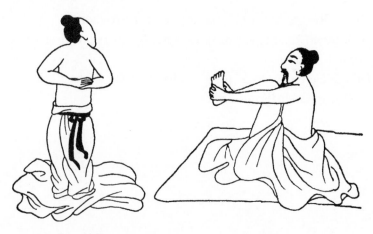

Figure 25.8   Figure 25.9

METHOD OF NOURISHING THE BLOOD

Application: Rheumatics, atrophy of hands and feet, and paralysis.

Method: While walking slowly, bend the elbows to lift the hands up and down. After a while, click the teeth. When the mouth is filled with saliva, swallow it. This exercise helps to nourish the blood, absorb internal humidity, ameliorate the function of the spleen and cure paralysis. (Figure 25.10)

METHOD OF REMAINING YOUNG

Application: Insufficient vital energy.

Method: Lie on the back, hold the left foot with the right hand and press the external sex organs with the left hand. This exercise helps to reinforce the vital energy and rejuvenate the body. (Figure 25.11)

METHOD OF REGULATING THE FUNCTIONS OF THE STOMACH

Application: Vomiting and diarrhea caused by upset stomach attacked by cold wind.

Method: Lie on the back, press one hand on the forehead and the other on the stomach. (Figure 25.12)

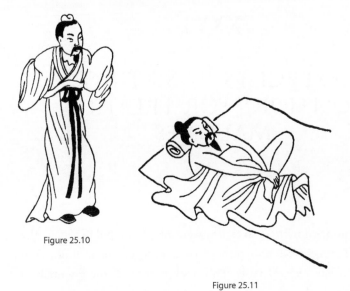

Figure 25.10

Figure 25.11

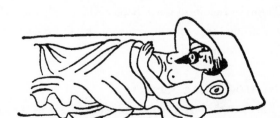

Figure 25.12

XXVI

Exercises in Sitting Positions for Treating Maladies

The illustrations for these exercises were originally published in the *Formulas of Exercises in Sitting Positions for Treating Maladies* by an anonymous writer of the late Qing Dynasty. This book introduces the essentials of ancient methods of *qigong* or *daoyin*. It originally contained 24 illustrations for the Exercises in Sitting Positions for Treating Maladies and 15 for the Daoyin of Xiaoyaozi (see Chapter XIV). Only the 1911 edition is extant, containing the 24 illustrations for the Exercises in Sitting Positions for Treating Maladies.

Overflow of two Sources

Sit with the legs straight, the heels close together and the toes pointing outwards. Bend and stretch the toes several times until you feel the warmth of the circulation *qi* at the acupuncture point Yongquan (about 1/3 of the way down from the toes on the sole of the foot). In this way, *yang* energy is produced under *yin* energy, and will circulate along the meridian of the

Jue-yin Liver on the feet, and then be directed towards the knees after passing through the lower legs. If *qi* does not pass this vital point, *yang* energy cannot rise, and the *yang* meridians will not be nourished. This exercise helps one avoid maladies and stay healthy. (Figure 26.1)

SHAKING THE KNEES LIKE A DRAGON

Practice this exercise in a sitting position at midnight. Place the hands on the ground behind you. Raise the knees, and separate and draw them together with a regular rhythm. Lead *qi* from the meridian of the Taiyin Spleen on the feet to the meridian of the Jueyin Liver, via the knees, finally arriving at the inner sides of the thighs. The feeling of formication is the sign that the exercise is taking effect. (Figure 26.2)

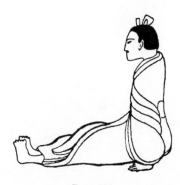

Figure 26.1

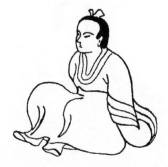

Figure 26.2

Beating the Mountain and the Valley

In a sitting position, slowly pound the legs with the fists from the knees along the outer sides of the thighs to the coccyx. Lead *qi* from the meridian of the Shaoyang Gall Bladder on the feet to the meridian of the Taiyin Spleen, also on the feet, and thence to the coccyx. (Figure 26.3)

Rubbing the Coccyx

In a sitting position, raise the external sex organs with the left hand, then blow on the right palm, and quickly move it behind the coccyx. Rub the coccyx with alternate hands. When practicing this exercise, close the eyes, roll the tongue, raise the shoulders and contract the muscles of the anus. Guide *qi* from the meridian of the Shaoyin Kidney on the feet to the meridian of the Shaoyang Gall Bladder. A straight warm current should rise from the coccyx to the head. The meridians are then unblocked. (Figure 26.4)

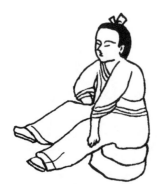

Figure 26.3

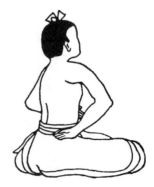

Figure 26.4

RAISING THE HANDS

In a standing position, raise the hands to chest level, then turn the palms to the sky as if you are supporting it. Thrust out the belly, and lean the head back, with the eyes fixed on the hands. After a while, lower the hands slowly to hang beside the body. When practicing this exercise, guide the breath to the *dantian* (in the lower abdomen). Raise the hands, and lead *qi* up to the head. Finally, allow *qi* to spread into the limbs so as to smooth all the meridians. (Figure 26.5)

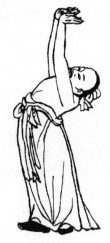

Figure 26.5

MASSAGING THE SPLEEN

Sit erect, rub the palms together until they become warm, and then quickly place them on the soft back part of each side of the vertebrae. Lead *qi* from the Taiyang Bladder meridian to the Shaoyin Kidney meridian. This is a very useful exercise for fortifying the essence of the body. (Figure 26.6)

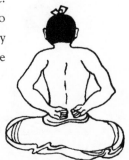

Figure 26.6

317

TURNING TWO WINDLASSES AT THE SAME TIME

Twirl the arms in unison from the shoulders about 20 or 30 times, as if you are turning two windlasses. Lead *qi* from the Yangming Stomach meridian on the feet to the nape of the neck and the Taiyang Bladder meridian on the feet. In this way, the renal fluid rises by itself with the *qi* and the blood. (Figure 26.7)

BENDING THE NECK

Sit erect, with the tip of the tongue touching the upper palate, and the eyes and mouth slightly closed. Bend the head towards the left 20 to 30 times, eyes looking to the left. Then repeat on the right side. Then suddenly shake the head with force, and contract the anal muscles once to lead *qi* to the top of the head. (Figure 26.8)

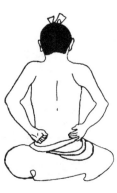

Figure 26.7

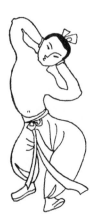

Figure 26.8

THE LION PULLS A TREE

Sit on a low stool, with the right leg extended. Grasp the right foot with the right hand. Kick with the right foot forcibly, and restrain it with the right hand. Repeat the movement on the other side. Lead *qi* from the Shaoyang Three Warmers (*sanjiao*) meridian to the Jueyin Pericardium meridian (both on the hands). In this way, the six *yang* meridians of the hands and the six *yin* meridians of the feet are linked every day. *Yin* and *yang qi* circulate freely in the body thanks to this exercise. (Figure 26.9)

FEROCIOUS TIGER'S STARE

Sit straight. Hold each shoulder with the opposite hand. Turn the head to the right, eyes staring fiercely like a tiger gazing at its prey. Then turn the body to the right and the head to the left, continuing the fierce stare. This exercise ameliorates the vision and dispels internal heat from the viscera. Bring *qi* from the meridian of the Large Intestine of Yangming on the hands to circulate in the meridian of Shaoyin Heart (also on the hands). (Figure 26.10)

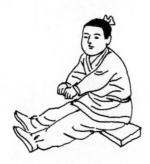
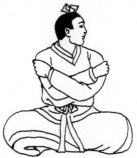

Figure 26.9   Figure 26.10

IMMORTAL CARRYING A SWORD

Sit straight, and raise the arms horizontally, inhaling so that the abdomen rises. Then bend the upper body toward the ground and return it to the erect position, raising the arms with force as if lifting a heavy load. Then slowly lower the arms to clasp the hands behind the back. In this way, *qi* and blood are allowed to circulate freely and vigorously, so as to eliminate stagnant *qi* in the heart or chest. (Figure 26.11)

DEMON BEATING A DRUM

Sit straight, with both fists clenched. Raise the fists as high as possible above the head. Then lower the fists as if pulling a heavy object down. Lead *qi* from the meridian of the Jueyin Pericardium on the hands to the meridian of the Small Intestine of Taiyang (also on the hands). (Figure 26.12)

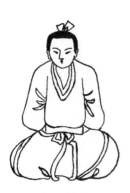 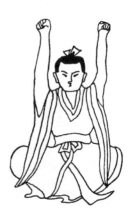

Figure 26.11   Figure 26.12

Young Disciple Fatigued by Salutation

Sit straight, with the legs together and straight out. Place one hand on each knee, elbows held to the sides, the mouth closed and the tongue rolled. Lower the head with force to the knees and spread the legs to the left and right, respectively. Lead *qi* from the meridian of the Small Intestine of Taiyin on the hands to the meridian of the Big Intestine of Yangming (also on the hands). This exercise is good for getting rid of leucoma and closing all the orifices of the vital organs in the body. (Figure 26.13)

Tornado Lion

Sit with the legs together and straight out. Lower the head, and incline the upper body. Then raise the body, holding the hands together in front of the chest. Turn the upper body to the left and then to the right. This exercise can help to harmonize the meridians and nurture the five viscera. (Figure 26.14)

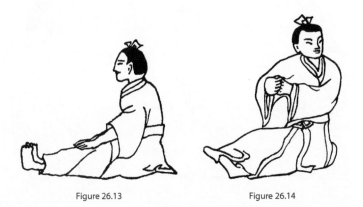

Figure 26.13   Figure 26.14

Waving a Stick in a Sack

Cross the arms and hold each elbow with the opposite hand. Turn the upper body alternately to the left and right. This exercise can help to unblock the meridians, warm the *dantian*, dispel stagnant *qi* and smooth the digestion. (Figure 26.15)

Shooting at Eagles on the Left and Right

Stand with the arms in the position of drawing a bow. Stretch the arms to the limit in order to make the blood and *qi* circulate freely in the limbs, instead of stagnating in the joints of the body. (Figure 26.16)

Sawing a Log

Stand still, and imitate a sawing movement, alternating to the left and right. This exercise can help to eliminate accumulated stagnant elements. (Figure 26.17)

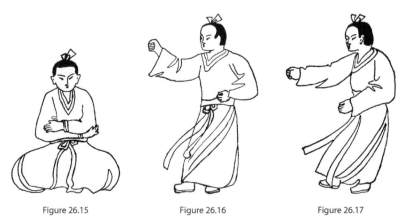

Figure 26.15   Figure 26.16   Figure 26.17

Dragon Extending its Claws

Sit straight, and raise both arms above the head as if you are supporting something. Lower the hands a little, and then lift them up again. Repeat this movement 15 times. Click the teeth, breathe and swallow the saliva. This exercise can treat the maladies caused by cold wind or other mild factors leading to illness. (Figure 26.18)

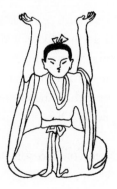

Figure 26.18

Playing the Flute

Sit straight, and regulate the breath. Then place both hands on the ground behind you. Stick out and suck in the belly alternately while inhaling and exhaling. Close the mouth, roll the tongue and stick out the belly until a warm feeling appears in it and there is a gurgling sound in the intestines. Then the problems of stagnation are solved. If you practice this exercise every day, stagnation can be dispelled and maladies cured. A moment later, regulate *qi* to unblock all meridians and internal organs. (Figure 26.19)

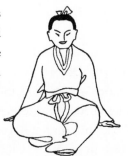

Figure 26.19

Tumbling of the Celestial Guardian

Hold the elbows with the opposite hands, putting the weight on the balls of the feet. Stamp hard with the heels. This exercise can reinforce the kidneys, and fortify *qi* and blood. (Figure 26.20)

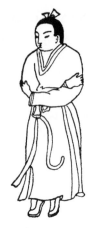

Figure 26.20

Moving the Tongue while Breathing

Sit on a stool, with the right foot placed on the left knee. Interlace the fingers, and sway the hands within the breadth of the shoulders back and forth 30 times. Then regulate the breath, concentrate the attention and move the tongue to the left and right in the mouth. Once the mouth is filled with saliva, swallow it in three swallows while making a sound. Then breathe out the waste air and regulate the breath. (Figure 26.21)

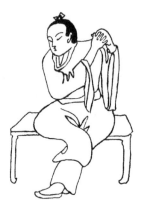

Figure 26.21

Clicking the Teeth and Beating the Celestial Drum

Sit straight, and click the teeth to concentrate the mind. Regulate the breath to nourish *qi*. Tap the occiput with the fingers to activate the *yin* essence in the body. Click the teeth again to stimulate the *yang* energy. The vital energy is thereby concentrated in the brain, helping to prolong life. (Figure 26.22)

MAKING THE SUN AND MOON TURN

After completing the previous exercise, a feeling of heat should emerge in all meridians and vessels of the body. You should then regulate the breath until it becomes soft and gentle. Slightly close the eyes, and slowly turn the eyeballs to the left and then to the right. This exercise can dispel "toxic fire" from the eyes and humidify them with kidney fluid. (Figure 26.23)

CLOSING THE MOUTH AND LOWERING THE CURTAIN

Sit straight, close the mouth and roll the tongue, with the eyes half closed. Focus the eyes on the nose and then on the *dantian*. Keep the spine straight, and allow the fluid in the kidneys to rise by itself. Concentrate the attention on the *dantian*. (Figure 26.24)

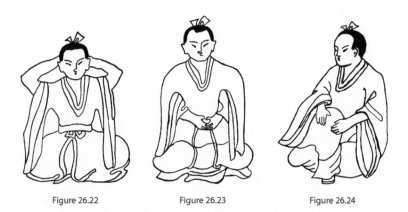

Figure 26.22   Figure 26.23   Figure 26.24